Guide to
Safe, Anxiety-Free
Dental Surgery

Jeffrey V. Anzalone, DDS

About The Author	7
Meet The Anzalones	9
Acknowledgments	11
Overview of the BIG PICTURE	13
The 9 Most Important Dental Surgery Secrets	13
Chapter 2 Selecting the Right Dental Surgeon	17
What Are the Dental Specialties That Perform Surgery?	19
What Is a Periodontist?	20
Chapter 3 The Consultation	23
The Initial Consultation: Examining the Doctor	25
Am I a candidate for surgery?	26
14 Questions to Ask Your Prospective Periodontist	27
Chapter 4 Gum Disease (Periodontitis)	29
Gum Disease Symptoms	30
Pocket Recording	32
Is gum disease contagious?	32
Gum Disease and the Human Body	33
Gum Disease and Cardiovascular Disease	33
Gum Disease and Other Systemic Diseases	34
Gum Disease and Women	35
Gum Disease and Children	37
Signs of Periodontal Disease	38
Advice for Parents	39
Gum Disease Risk Factors	41
Non-Surgical Periodontal Treatment	42
Regenerative Procedures	43
Pocket Reduction Procedures	44
Follow-Up Care	45
Chapter 5 The Photo Gallery	47
Free Gingival Graft	47
Connective Tissue Graft	49
Dental Implants	51
Sinus Lift With Dental Implant Placement	53
Classification of Implant Sites	53
Implants placed after sinus has been elevated	54

Sinus Lift as a Separate Procedure · 55
Sinus Perforation · 55
Bone Grafting · 57
Esthetic Crown Lengthening · 59
Crown Lengthening for a Restoration · 60
Tooth Extraction and Socket Grafting · 61
More Photos of Procedures · 62
Connective Tissue Graft · 62
Connective Tissue Graft + Crowns · 64
Free Gingival Graft · 64
Esthetic Crown Lengthening · 65
Crown Lengthening for a Restoration · 67

Chapter 6 Dental Implants · 69
Bridge Versus Implant · 70
Dental Bridge · 71
Repair or Replace? · 72
Fixed Restoration · 76
Removable Restoration · 76
Bonus Section for Denture Wearers · 81

Chapter 7 Sedation Dentistry · 83
Anesthesia Choices · 84
Chapter 8 Aftercare · 89
Typical Recovery Times · 89
What the Top Periodontists Do to Speed Your Recovery · 89

Chapter 9 Erasing Mental Blocks · 91

Chapter 10 The Relationship Between Your Dentist and Your Periodontist · 95
Why can't my dentist treat me? · 95
Can my dentist treat my gum disease? · 95
Why do I have to go to another office for an implant? · 97

About The Author

Jeffrey V. Anzalone, DDS, is a board certified periodontist in Monroe, La. He was born and raised in Monroe and decided his hometown was the perfect place to raise his family. Dr. Anzalone attended Northeast Louisiana University and is a graduate of Louisiana State University Dental School.

After dental school, Dr. Anzalone completed a one-year General Practice Residency at the VA Medical Center in Biloxi, Miss., and one year of private practice in general dentistry before deciding to return to LSU for specialty training. He completed his specialty residency training in periodontics at Louisiana State University in New Orleans. Dr. Anzalone is a Diplomate of the American Board of Periodontology. A Diplomate is a periodontist who has made significant achievements beyond the mandatory educational requirements of the specialty and who is certified by the American Board of Periodontology. This optional certification demonstrates a dentist's commitment to providing excellent dental care to patients.

Dr. Anzalone is active within his professional community, working to promote best practices in patient care. Dr. Anzalone is the author of *What They Don't Teach You In Dental School*, a book written to help young dentists who are just starting their practices to focus on serving their patients well. He also writes several monthly newsletters and has published a case study in the Journal of Oral Implantology.

Dr. Anzalone had no plans for specializing in periodontics until the specialty first piqued his interest while he was in his residency at the VA Medical Center. Like most students, he was ready to graduate and begin earning a living. Instead, he followed his true passion and continued his education so he could practice the type of dentistry he had come to love. Now he wouldn't change that decision for anything. Dr. Anzalone not only enjoys treating his patients, but he also invests many hours of his time into staying up-todate in the profession by attending numerous continuing education seminars each year. He also speaks at these events, teaching other dentists what is working in his practice so they, too, can deliver top-notch patient care.

Meet the Anzalone's

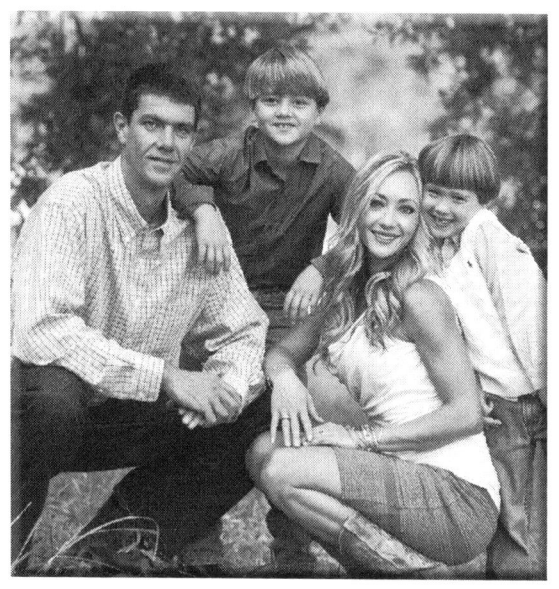

Jeffrey, Brooks (7), Rebekah, and Benton (5)

Acknowledgments

I could write an entire book about the numerous people I should thank for helping me get to the position I am in today. To my wife and best friend, Rebekah, not only are you the love of my life, but you are also my rock and support. To my wonderful little boys, Brooks and Benton, you guys keep what's important in life in perspective. To my parents, Frank and Patsy, thank you for raising me right in a wrong world. To all my colleagues and to Dan Kennedy for all the marketing wisdom, I will always be grateful.Thank you to all.

The computer-generated pictures in *Everything You Need to Know About Dental Surgery* are from the Consult Pro software program.

Overview of the
BIG PICTURE

Considering Dental Surgery?
- Is it difficult to decide which doctor to choose?
- Would you like to know the step-by-step process?
- Do you need some help to make your decision?
- Are you wondering why your family dentist can't treat you?
- Are you frightened by the unknowns?
- Would you like to have an insider's view of the entire process from start to finish?

If yes is your answer to any or all of the above questions, then I have good news for you. The book you are holding in your hands addresses all these questions and much, much more.

I'd like to begin by sharing with you my nine most important secrets about dental surgery:

The 9 Most Important Dental Surgery Secrets

Secret #1. All dentists can perform dental surgery, but many lack the proper training.

Secret #2. The surgeon should be able to provide a "before" and an "after" album at your request.

Secret #3. DO YOUR HOMEWORK. Choosing a dentist that performs the type of surgical procedure you require is difficult.

Secret #4. The consultation appointment should focus on teaching you about the treatment options, not on "selling" you on a particular procedure.

Secret #5. Knowing the right questions to ask your periodontist will help you make the best decisions about your treatment.

Secret #6. Fees are negotiable. Don't be afraid to ask.

Secret #7. The office facility where your treatment will be performed is as important as the dentist performing the treatment.

Secret #8. Learning about "aftercare" before surgery will help decrease post-surgical complications.

Secret #9. Low fees are not always a bargain.

High fees do not always ensure the best results. Yes, I know what you are thinking now: I need to obtain and process a lot of information before my first appointment! But remember, most periodontal and implant surgery is elective and is not for everyone. You and your dentist should consider multiple factors, including your overall health, before deciding on surgery. A doctor and a patient should be on the same page, and this book will give you the specific information you need to make a confident decision.

One of the most important decisions will be selecting your doctor. More than likely, your general dentist will refer you to a specialist that he or she believes is right for you. If you are not comfortable with that doctor and/or staff, you should consider other options.

I love what I do for a living, but sometimes I need to advise a patient not to have surgery, even when the general dentist has recommended it.

> *"I like the fact that everyone at Anzalone Periodontics was professional, courteous, polite, and understanding." — Lenora Lawhon (wife of Todd Lawhon, DDS)*

For example, I may believe the person's health would make the procedure too risky. In that case, I would make recommendations to help decrease the risk before considering treatment.

Just for fun, I googled the search term "dental surgery" and obtained more than 23 million search results. Yes, you read that correctly, 23 million. In my opinion, there is TOO MUCH information available from too many different sources, especially on the internet. Most of it confuses rather than educates.

Because of the enormous amount of information available, my goal is to:
- Give you information that is very important for your decision making (information that many dentists and specialists may not tell you.
- Share with you the best ways to become self-educated about selecting your doctor and treatment options.
- Provide you with step-by-step instructions to begin your journey through the "minefield" of information available.

Chapter 2
Selecting the Right Dental Surgeon

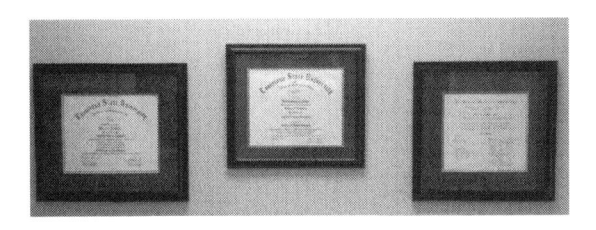

Secret: DO YOUR HOMEWORK. Selecting a dentist that performs the type of surgical procedure you require is difficult.

For the most part, dental surgery is elective. Certainly there are some occasions when infection or another medical problem poses a danger to a person's health that requires immediate attention. But for the most part, dental surgical procedures can be put on hold to allow you to gather valuable information to make the best decision possible. Should your general dentist treat you? Should you see a specialist? Can your friend's dentist treat you? What if the dentist is old? Is it a good sign if he or she drives an expensive car? Some of the answers to these questions may surprise you.

Most patients are referred for surgical care to a dental specialist by their family dentist. Dentists see firsthand the type of work a surgeon performs, so they are an excellent information source. Other referral sources are family members and friends that have been pleased with their surgical outcomes. The amount of information may be overwhelming when you are deciding whom to choose, so you may want to start with this basic list of criteria:

1. **Graduation from a recognized school of dentistry**
2. **Completion of an accredited residency recognized by the American Dental Association (ADA)**
3. **State dental license in the state where the dentist practices**
4. **Board certification** - A board certified dental specialist denotes someone who has made significant achievements beyond the mandatory educational requirements of the specialty. Mastering a series of written and oral exams is required to obtain this credential. Each board usually establishes and enforces a recertification requirement.

> *"I was referred to Dr. Anzalone from my regular dentist. I had some periodontal problems that had been going on for quite a while. Dr. Anzalone looked at the situation, performed treatment on me, and I am very well pleased. I am pleased with the results, the very caring staff, and I would recommend him to anyone that needs that type of treatment." — Pat L*

What Are the Dental Specialties That Perform Surgery?
The answer to the above question may shock you. Just about all of the specialties perform some type of dental surgery, including general dentists. The specialties are:

- Endodontist - Performs root canal therapy, diagnosis, and treatment of other diseases and injuries to the pulp or soft tissue of the tooth. Some also place dental implants.
- Oral Surgeon - Diagnoses and operates on disease, injuries, and defects in the mouth, jaw, and face. Also places dental implants.
- Prosthodontist - Treats patients with simple to complex conditions associated with missing or deficient teeth. Also places dental implants.

Removing a tooth that involves cutting of the gum tissue and/or bone is considered a surgery. For the remainder of this book and to help keep things as simple as possible, when dental surgery is mentioned, we are speaking of periodontal (gum) and dental implant surgery that is performed by a periodontist.

> *"I was referred to Dr. Anzalone from my dentist for an extraction and an implant. I had concerns about the treatment due to my age, 85 years. Dr. Anzalone performed the procedure at minimal discomfort to me. I loved his personal care towards me and very much appreciated his telephone calls the afternoon and evening after my procedure.*
> *He is #1 in my book!"* — Fred Westrom

What Is a Periodontist?

The answer to this question was taken directly from the American Academy of Periodontology's website:

A periodontist is a dentist who specializes in the prevention, diagnosis, and treatment of periodontal disease, and in the placement of dental implants. Periodontists are also experts in the treatment of oral inflammation. Periodontists receive extensive training in these areas, including three additional years of education beyond dental school. They are familiar with the latest techniques for diagnosing and treating periodontal disease, and are also trained in performing cosmetic periodontal procedures.

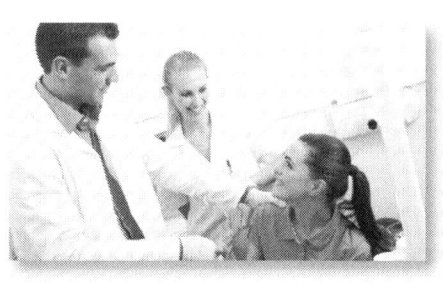

Periodontal Treatments

Periodontists often treat more problematic periodontal cases, such as those with severe gum disease or a complex medical history. Periodontists offer a wide range of treatments, such as scaling and root planing (in which the infected surface of the root is cleaned) or root surface debridement (in which damaged tissue is removed). They can also treat patients with severe gum problems, using a range of surgical procedures. In addition, periodontists are specially trained in the placement and repair of dental implants.

Specialty Overlap

Specialty overlap is when two or more specialties are equally capable of performing the same procedures. The two main areas of overlap are dental extractions with or without bone grafting and dental implant surgery. As of this writing, the main dental specialties that perform both of these types of treatment are periodontists, prosthodontists, and oral surgeons.

As you may imagine, there have been "turf battles" between overlapping specialties. This is also a major issue in medicine among plastic surgeons, dermatologists, head and neck surgeons, and ophthalmologists with regard to peforming cosmetic surgery.

Doctor Selection
More than likely your dentist will suggest a doctor to perform your surgery. It is your job to take the information you are holding in your hands to make an informed decision. Since you are the final decision maker, remember to slow down and take your time to process the information you learn here and from others who have visited the prospective doctor.

You should receive educational materials from the surgeon, before your initial visit, regarding the office, staff, doctor, and your treatment options. Your potential surgeon's experience is of primary importance. The procedure you are considering should be one the surgeon routinely performs, so always ask how many procedures of the type you are considering the doctor performs each month or year.

The office decor and staff can also tell you a lot about the doctor. Top professionals surround themselves with top-notch staff. But dental surgery is not glamorous, so don't become enamored with the office decor. Your mouth is more important that the type of couch in the waiting area. Also, evaluate the doctor's personality:

- Does he or she display a positive attitude?
- Is he or she friendly to you?
- Is he or she friendly to the staff?
- Does he or she seem pleased with or annoyed by your questions?

Should I rely on advertisements?
We are inundated daily by advertisements on radio, TV, email, newspaper, and magazines. Did you know that the average person comes in contact with more than 3,000 advertisements daily?

My response regarding advertisements is this: Does the ad try to teach you something? Advertisements that focus solely on selling fail to educate and sometimes mislead the prospective patient.

An ad that focuses on teaching you about a procedure or that tells a story about a patient's recent experience will help you make a more educated decision.

You may be asking yourself, "Why should a dentist have to advertise?" Perhaps you immediately distrust professionals such as attorneys, physicians, and financial advisors that advertise. This type of thinking can be counterproductive. As a matter of fact, I found most of the professionals I work with through their advertisements. If I hadn't seen their ads, I might have never benefited from their services!

The more these professionals perform their work, the better their work is. (Practice makes perfect.) Advertising their services keeps them busy. Who wants to go to a surgeon who rarely operates and is likely on the golf course every afternoon? I don't, and I know you don't either.

Some people treat professionals that advertise with disdain. They think a professional's reputation should be so ironclad and well known that advertising is unnecessary. Consider this: Most people who purchase an expensive car or a fine piece of jewelry are usually motivated at least somewhat by an advertisement. High-end companies such as Lexus, Rolls Royce, and Tiffany's advertise their quality products. What makes them any different from a dentist doing the same? Large companies recognize the value of their services and products, and they also recognize the value of advertising to a larger audience. So do professionals, like dentists. Enough said.

> *"Dr. Anzalone's staff was friendly, direct, and very pleasant."* — *Paul Cobum*

Chapter 3
The Consultation

Secret: The consultation appointment should teach you about the treatment options. It should not be focused solely on selling.

The Initial Consultation: Examining the Doctor It has probably been several years since you took a school exam, but this test should be easy. The answers to all your questions and concerns lie in your hands. Think of this examination as an open book test, which most people pass with flying colors. After thoroughly studying this book, you will be able to ask intelligent questions about your recommended treatment—and the doctor.

Have you heard the phrase "You only get one chance to make a first impression"? In someperiodontal offices, the initial consultation is with a staff member such as a hygienist or a dental assistant, and then the financial coordinator is brought in to "close" the deal. The doctor may stop in for a brief "hello" and then disappears. This scenario happens time and time again and does not leave a good first impression.

The Initial Phone Call
I can still recall a phone conversation I had some years ago. Although I don't frequent many doctors' offices, I do know how a call with a prospective patient (me) should be handled. Upon calling the office, I was greeted by a gruff, impatient voice that immediately placed me on hold (without asking). After several minutes of holding and hearing a loud beeping sound, the call resumed. My contact information was obtained and an appointment was given. I was not given any time to ask questions; the call ended as quickly as it had begun.

Needless to say, this doctor lost his prospective patient before the initial visit. Here are my criteria you can use to judge the initial phone call:

- The call is answered within three or four rings — you should never get a busy signal.
- A cheerful, warm staff member greets you with a "good morning" or "good afternoon."
- Your questions are answered by someone with a helpful and caring attitude.
- If a staff member cannot answer your questions, you are promptly connected with someone who can.
- Before your initial visit, the office sends you complimentary booklets, brochures, DVDs, audio CDs, etc. These materials should carefully explain the different types of procedures the doctor performs. Becoming educated about the dental procedures will help you make the best decision possible regarding your treatment options.
- The staff member works with your schedule to provide a suitable date and time for the appointment.
- Patient registration forms are either mailed or offered online to be filled out before the initial consultation to help expedite the appointment.
- A copy of the office's financial policy is also provided beforehand. An exact fee quotation requires the doctor's examination and an evaluation of any X-rays brought or taken. A superior dental office will offer a broad range of fees for the procedure(s) in which you are interested.
- The office informs you that you will be contacted one day prior to the appointment as a reminder and also to answer any other questions that may arise.
- The practice's web address is given for additional information such as a map or driving directions to the office's location.

When scheduling the consultation, the more information you can provide about your desires the better. For instance, if you have had unsuccessful surgery in the past or a bad experience with a previous periodontist, please inform the staff member. This will allow the staff member to ask different questions to personalize your care. For example, previous dental records may need to be obtained before your consultation. Having this information will help the doctor to decide the right treatment options for you.

You may be thinking to yourself that this is a lot of information to give and receive before arriving at the office. As stated before, you should expect exceptional customer service, and this begins with the initial phone call. If the doctor and the staff are not competent and particular about details up front, how competent will they be while treating you?

The Initial Consultation

Have you ever eaten at a restaurant and noticed that the floors and tables were dirty? Can you imagine what the kitchen looked like? We use our five senses to judge our surroundings, and sight is one of the most important. So, evaluate how the dental office looks. It should be neat, clean, and devoid of any litter. If not, what can you expect about the condition of the surgical instruments and tools that will be used in your mouth?

Upon arriving at the office, a warm, friendly staff member should greet you. A good surgical practice is more than just the services from the doctor. The practice should be staffed with competent, top-notch staff members to facilitate meeting all the needs of their patients. You should feel more like a "guest" than a patient.

If you did not fill out medical forms prior to your visit, you will be given some to complete. In addition, X-ray films may need to be taken before you consult with the doctor. The staff should review your medical history and ask questions regarding your visit. Then it will be time to meet with the doctor.

The interview with the doctor should be relaxed and informative. He or she will review your medical history and ask questions pertinent to your desires. He or she should use nonmedical terms when discussing treatment options as well as visual aids either in book or video form to help clarify exactly what is involved with the treatment. The doctor should answer any questions you have with patience and frankness. Not only does the doctor need to determine if you are a good candidate for treatment, but you, too, should determine if it's the right thing for you.

Occasionally, a multiphased treatment plan is needed to bring a patient's mouth back to health. This will require not only surgical treatment, but also care from the patient's family dentist. In this situation, the periodontist will consult with the referring dentist to discuss the best treatment options and then have the patient back for a reconsultation. At times, treatment between the two offices will need to be coordinated since both offices may need to see the patient on the same day. The more time you spend discussing your options before the surgery, the clearer the overall picture will become.

Am I a candidate for surgery?

With more and more patients taking prescription medicines for health issues, it's especially important that both the staff and the doctor review the medical history. Certain medications (e.g., blood thinners) will need to be discontinued before treatment, and consulting with the patient's physician is required.

Local anesthetic agents commonly used by dentists cause the blood pressure and pulse to rise. For this reason, blood pressure readings must be taken before the administration of these agents. Our office routinely diagnoses patients with hypertension and refers them to their family physician to get the condition under control before treating them. The motto in the periodontist's office should be Safety First.

"I want to express my gratitude to you for your excellent professional care of my family and me." — Connie Ward

14 Questions to Ask Your Prospective Periodontist

How many times have you left a doctor's office and then remembered the question you meant to ask? It's sometimes difficult to think of all the possible questions concerning treatment in one appointment. These 14 questions will keep you on track:

1. How long have you been performing the type of procedure I am considering? How many do you perform a year?
2. Am I a good candidate for the proposed treatment?
3. What type of anesthesia do you offer?
4. Where will the surgery take place?
5. How long will it take to complete the surgery?
6. How painful is it after surgery?
7. When can I return to work/school?
8. How long is the entire treatment period (surgery, recovery, and any necessary followup)?
9. Will I be given a written estimate for treatment?
10. Will you file my dental insurance and provide all supporting documents and X-rays?
11. Do you have payment plans, preferably with interest-free options?
12. Are you board certified?
13. Have you written books or journal articles on periodontal surgery?
14. Do you lecture at continuing education events and educate your referring dentist colleagues?

So, how will you know if the doctor and the staff have given you the correct answers to the above questions? By the time you complete reading this book, you will recognize each correct answer when you hear it.

Secret: The surgeon should provide a "before" and "after" album at your request.

The human mind learns best with pictures. If I say the word "elephant," what comes to mind? The word *elephant* or the picture of an elephant? Probably the latter. That is why your treatment options should not only be explained, but also shown with pictures. A good "before" and "after" album will help you get a sense of the outcome to expect.

I'm amazed when I learn that patients who have visited other offices were never given a chance to look at this type of album. Would you build or remodel a house before reviewing work your potential contractor has performed? I think not, and your dental work should be no different.

Chapter 4
Gum Disease
(Periodontitis)

One of every two American adults age 30 and over has periodontal disease, according to recent findings from the Centers for Disease Control and Prevention (CDC). A study titled <u>Prevalence of Periodontitis in Adults in the United States: 2009 and 2010</u> estimates that 47.2 percent, or 64.7 million American adults, have mild, moderate, or severe gum disease (periodontitis). In adults 65 and older, prevalence rates increase to 70.1 percent. This study is published in the Journal of Dental Research, the official publication of the International and American Associations for Dental Research.

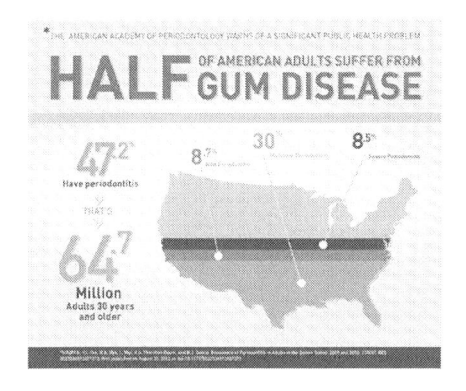

Mr. Bill's Story:

"How can this happen? How can I have gum disease if I brush my teeth every day?" This was Mr. Bill's response after my consultation. I informed him that unfortunately most gum disease is not painful and he may have had this condition for years without knowing it.

Periodontal disease is a low-grade chronic bacterial infection and the number one cause of tooth loss. While everyone has bacteria in their mouth, not everyone develops gum disease. There are identifiable risk factors that can make it more likely for the bacteria in your mouth to result in destructive gum disease. We now know that due to these risk factors, some patients can clean their teeth and visit the dentist religiously and still have gum problems.

Over time, bacteria tend to collect between the teeth and gum. If this debris is not adequately removed, the bacteria migrate deeper under the gum line. In a susceptible patient, a space or "pocket" forms between the tooth and the gum. Once these pockets of bacteria form below the gum line, you cannot reach them—even with good brushing and flossing.

The bacteria multiply and cause the gum cells to release a variety of substances that aggravate and inflame the gum tissues. The gum tissue and then the supporting bone are slowly destroyed. If enough bone tissue is destroyed, the teeth loosen and are eventually lost.

Gum Disease Symptoms

Periodontal disease rarely causes pain or any symptoms since the infection readily drains up through the gum. Often you cannot tell you have gum disease until the gum is inspected and checked for pockets. It's like having termites in your house. Above the ground the house looks fine, but the foundation is slowly being destroyed without you knowing it.

It's the same way with gum disease. Just because it doesn't hurt doesn't mean all is well. But we do not need to wait until damage has been done to tell if you have gum disease. Gum disease can be detected early and its damage repaired.

You can also keep watch. Bleeding is a strong indicator of gum inflammation. Healthy gums do not bleed at all when brushed or flossed. If you have any gum bleeding when you clean your teeth, your gums are inflamed. Other symptoms include: gums that are receding or pulling away from the teeth, causing the teeth to look longer than before; loose or separating teeth; pus between your teeth and gums; sores in your mouth; persistent bad breath; and a change in the way your teeth fit together when you bite.

> *"You and your staff made me feel so comfortable during my teeth extraction appointment. It was a lot LESS painful than I was expecting. You guys explained everything step by step. I work with patients myself and know how important it is to explain the procedures to patients. Thanks again for making me comfortable and caring for me." — William Lansing*

Pocket Recording

Pocket recording is a way we can assess the condition of your gums. The following graphic explains the procedure:

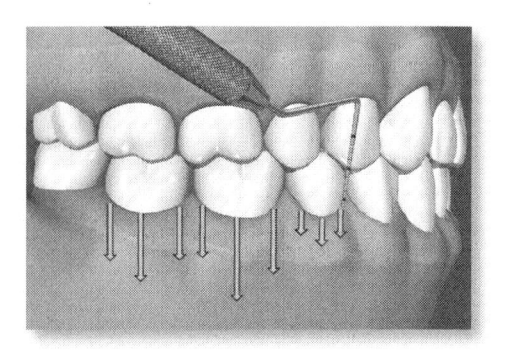

Periodontal pocketing is measured with a special instrument called a periodontal probe. It has 1 millimeter markings engraved on it. The pocket depths are recorded in three locations in front of and behind the tooth for a total of six readings. These pocket depths along with X-rays help the dentist determine the amount of bone loss a person has.

Is gum disease contagious?

Research has shown that periodontal disease is caused by the inflammatory reaction to bacteria under the gums, so periodontal disease technically may not be contagious. However, the bacteria that cause the inflammatory reaction can be spread through saliva. This means that if one of your family members has periodontal disease, it's a good idea to avoid contact with his or her saliva by not sharing eating utensils or oral health equipment. If you notice that your spouse or a family member has the warning signs of a possible periodontal problem (bleeding, red and swollen gums, or bad breath), you may want to suggest that he or she sees a periodontist for an exam. It may help to protect the oral health of everyone in the family.

Gum Disease and the Human Body

We now know that an ongoing bacterial infection in your mouth can have far-reaching effects elsewhere in your body. When the gums are chronically inflamed, bacteria can gain entrance into your bloodstream and spread to other parts of your body. Gum disease increases your risk for diseases such as diabetes, cardiovascular disease, respiratory disease, osteoporosis, and cancer.

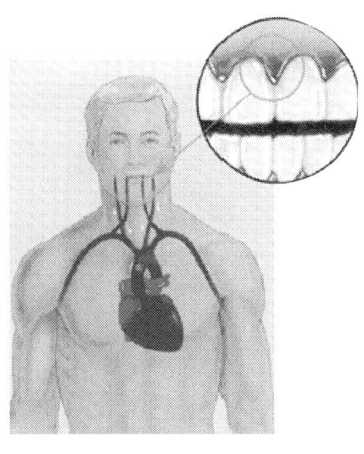

Gum Disease and Diabetes

Diabetic patients are more likely to develop periodontal disease, which in turn can increase blood sugar and diabetic complications. People with diabetes are more likely to have periodontal disease than people without diabetes, probably because people with diabetes are more susceptible to contracting infections. In fact, periodontal disease is often considered a complication of diabetes. People who don't have their diabetes under control are especially at risk.

Research has suggested that the relationship between periodontal disease and diabetes goes both ways—periodontal disease may make it more difficult for people who have diabetes to Severe periodontal disease can increase blood sugar, contributing to increased periods of time when the body functions with a high blood sugar. This puts people with diabetes at increased risk for diabetic complications.

Gum Disease and Cardiovascular Disease
Heart Disease

Several studies have shown that periodontal disease is associated with heart disease. While a cause-and-effect relationship has not yet been proven, research has indicated that periodontal disease increases the risk of heart disease.

Scientists believe that inflammation caused by periodontal disease may be responsible for the association.

Periodontal disease can also exacerbate existing heart conditions. Patients at risk for infective endocarditis may require antibiotics prior to dental procedures. Your periodontist and cardiologist will be able to determine if your heart condition requires use of antibiotics prior to dental procedures.

Stroke
Additional studies have pointed to a relationship between periodontal disease and stroke. In one study that looked at the causal relationship of oral infection as a risk factor for stroke, people diagnosed with acute cerebrovascular ischemia (stroke) were found more likely to have an oral infection when compared to those in the control group.

Gum Disease and Other Systemic Diseases
Osteoporosis
Researchers have suggested a link between osteoporosis (low bone mineral density) and bone loss in the jaw. Studies suggest that osteoporosis may lead to tooth loss because the density of the bone that supports the teeth may be decreased, which means the teeth no longer have a solid foundation.

Respiratory Disease
Bacteria that grow in the oral cavity can be aspirated into the lungs and cause respiratory diseases such as pneumonia, especially in people with periodontal disease.

Cancer
Researchers have found that men with gum disease were 49 percent more likely to develop kidney cancer, 54 percent more likely to develop pancreatic cancer, and 30 percent more likely to develop blood cancers.

"Thanks for making it possible to have my two front teeth for Christmas. I just may be the oldest patient you have. Thanks for your great work!" — *Dub Jones (former NFL player and father to Bert Jones)*

Gum Disease and Women

A woman's periodontal health may be impacted by a variety of factors.

Puberty

During puberty, an increased level of sex hormones, such as progesterone and possibly estrogen, causes increased blood circulation to the gums. This may cause an increase in the gums' sensitivity and lead to a greater reaction to any irritation, including food particles and plaque. During this time, the gums may become swollen, turn red, and feel tender.

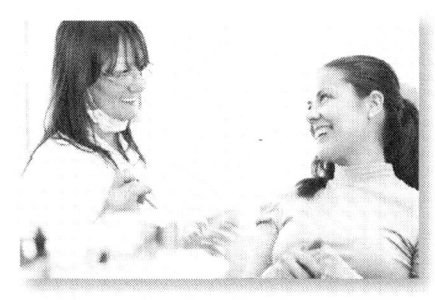

Menstruation

Occasionally, some women experience menstruation gingivitis. Women with this condition may experience bleeding gums, bright red and swollen gums, and sores on the inside of the cheek. Menstruation gingivitis typically occurs right before a woman's period and clears up once her period has started.

Pregnancy

Some studies have suggested the possibility of an additional risk factor in pregnancy — periodontal disease. Pregnant women who have periodontal disease may be more likely to have a baby that is born too early and too small. However, more research is needed to confirm how periodontal disease may affect pregnancy outcomes.

All infections are cause for concern among pregnant women because they pose a risk to the health of the baby. The American Academy of Periodontology now recommends that women considering pregnancy have a periodontal evaluation.

Menopause and Post-Menopause

Women who are menopausal or postmenopausal may experience changes in their mouth. They may notice discomfort in the mouth, including dry mouth, pain and burning sensations in the gum tissue, and altered taste, especially salty, peppery, or sour.

In addition, menopausal gingivostomatitis affects a small percentage of women. Gums that look dry or shiny, bleed easily, and range from abnormally pale to deep red mark this condition. Most women find that estrogen supplements help to relieve these symptoms.

> *"I was referred for dental implants and initially did not know what to expect with implants. The staff and Dr. Anzalone walked me through each step of the way and were very friendly. I never had to wait, and they explained all procedures very well."* — *Sonya Fuller*

Gum Disease and Children

> ***Jonathon's Story***
> *Jonathon's dentist called me to give me a "heads up" regarding his condition. Jonathon was 18 years old and wanted to get his teeth straightened. The orthodontist became alarmed after evaluating his X-rays and finding a significant amount of bone loss and loose teeth. Jonathon's mom was frantic and couldn't understand how this could have happened to her son. Unfortunately, Jonathon lost several teeth during the course of his many treatments, but those teeth were eventually replaced after the resolution of his aggressive form of gum disease.*

Types of Periodontal Diseases in Children

- Chronic gingivitis is common in children. It usually causes gum tissue to swell, turn red, and bleed easily. Gingivitis is both preventable and treatable with a regular routine of brushing, flossing, and professional dental care. However, left untreated, it can eventually advance to more serious forms of periodontal disease.
- Aggressive periodontitis can affect young people who are otherwise healthy. Localized aggressive periodontitis is found in teenagers and young adults and mainly affects the first molars and incisors. It is characterized by the severe loss of alveolar (jaw) bone, and ironically, patients generally form very little dental plaque or calculus (tartar).
- Generalized aggressive periodontitis may begin around puberty and involve the entire mouth. It is marked by inflammation of the gums and heavy accumulations of plaque and calculus. Eventually it can cause the teeth to become loose.

> *"I like the relaxed yet professional atmosphere of the office and staff, and I really appreciated the comfort during and after the implant treatment." —Scott Brown, DDS*

Signs of Periodontal Disease
Four basic signs will alert you to periodontal disease in your child:

1. Bleeding
Bleeding gums during tooth brushing, flossing, or at any other time.

2. Puffiness
Swollen and bright red gums

3. Recession
Gums that have receded away from the teeth, sometimes exposing the roots.

4. Bad breath
Constant bad breath that does not clear up with brushing and flossing.

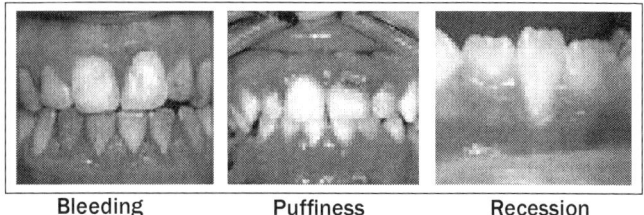

Bleeding　　　　Puffiness　　　　Recession

Importance of Good Dental Hygiene in Adolescents
Hormonal changes related to puberty can put teens at greater risk for getting periodontal disease. During puberty, an increased level of hormones, such as progesterone and possibly estrogen, cause increased blood circulation to the gums. This may cause an increase in the gums' sensitivity and lead to a greater reaction to any irritation, including food particles and plaque. During this time, the gums may become swollen, turn red, and feel tender.

As a teen progresses through puberty, the tendency for the gums to swell in response to irritants will lessen. However, during puberty, it is very important to follow a good at-home dental hygiene regimen, including regular brushing and flossing, and regular dental care. In some cases, a dental professional may recommend periodontal therapy to help prevent damage to the tissues and bone surrounding the teeth.

Advice for Parents

Early diagnosis is important for successful treatment of periodontal diseases. Therefore, it is important that children receive a comprehensive periodontal examination as part of their routine dental visits. Be aware that if your child has an advanced form of periodontal disease, this may be an early sign of systemic disease. A general medical evaluation should be considered for children who exhibit severe periodontitis, especially if it appears resistant to therapy.

The most important preventive step against periodontal disease is to establish good oral health habits with your child. Here are basic preventive steps to help your child maintain good oral health:

1. Establish good dental hygiene habits early. When your child is 12 months old, you can begin using toothpaste when brushing his or her teeth. When the gaps between your child's teeth close, it's important to start flossing.
2. Serve as a good role model by practicing good dental hygiene habits yourself.
3. Schedule regular dental visits for family checkups, periodontal evaluations, and cleanings.
4. Check your child's mouth for the signs of periodontal disease, including bleeding gums, swollen and bright red gums, gums that are receding away from the teeth, and bad breath.

The progression of gum disease can be halted if the bacteria and debris are removed from the pockets in the gums. In years past, traditional gum treatment consisted of cutting away the diseased gum with the hope that the remaining tissue would heal and be healthy. Fortunately, a variety of new techniques have allowed us to treat chronic gum infections much more conservatively. Removing large amounts of diseased gum and then "packing" the gums is a thing of the past.

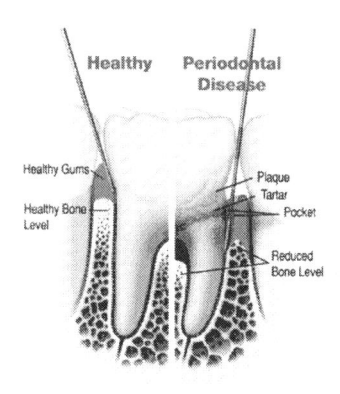

There are many forms of periodontitis. The most common ones include the following:

Aggressive periodontitis occurs in patients who are otherwise clinically healthy. Common features include rapid loss of tooth attachment and bone destruction, and this condition tends to run in families (familial aggregation).

Chronic periodontitis results in inflammation within the supporting tissues of the teeth, progressive loss of tooth attachment, and bone loss. This is the most frequently occurring form of periodontitis and is characterized by pocket formation and/or recession of the gingiva (gum). It is prevalent in adults, but can occur at any age. Progression of attachment loss usually occurs slowly, but periods of rapid progression can occur.

Periodontitis as a manifestation of systemic diseases often begins at a young age.

Necrotizing periodontal disease is an infection characterized by necrosis (death) of gingival tissues, periodontal ligament, and alveolar (jaw) bone. These lesions are most commonly observed in individuals with systemic conditions such as HIV infection, malnutrition, and immunosuppression.

Comprehensive Periodontal Evaluation

If gum disease is suspected, appropriate X-ray films will be taken to evaluate if bone loss exists around the teeth. Next, you should expect a comprehensive periodontal evaluation to take place. This evaluation is a way to assess your periodontal health by examining your teeth, gum tissue, plaque (bacteria) around the teeth, bite, bone structure, and risk factors.

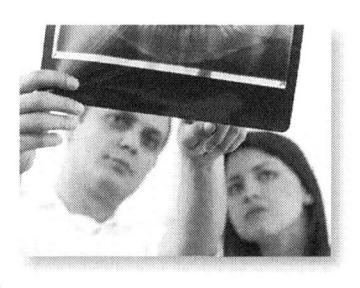

Gum Disease Risk Factors

- Age - The older you are, the higher your chances of acquiring gum disease. Data from the Centers for Disease Control and Prevention indicate that over 70 percent of Americans 65 and older have gum disease.
- Smoking/tobacco use - This is a two-fold problem. The first problem is that smokers with gum disease tend to lose bone up to three times faster versus nonsmokers. The second problem is that smokers do not respond as well to gum disease treatments versus nonsmokers.
- Clenching or grinding teeth - The excessive force this process causes on teeth also speeds up the rate at which the tissue supporting the teeth is destroyed.
- Stress - We are all under some type of stress. Research demonstrates that stress can make it more difficult for the body to fight off infection, including periodontal diseases.

"I was very fearful that my gum disease surgery might not be successful and that the pain and infection might return. I had been fighting gum disease (with my general dentist's help) for over a year. The pain was persistent and extreme for the month prior to treatment. Dr. Anzalone did a wonderful job, my problem was resolved, and I am NO LONGER suffering from painful gums. The surgery itself was much better than anticipated." — Jean Hibbard

You may be asking yourself, "What are my treatment options if I am diagnosed with gum disease?" Great question! The different treatments and procedures are discussed on the following pages.

Non-Surgical Periodontal Treatment
Periodontal health should be achieved in the least invasive and most cost-effective manner. This is often accomplished through non-surgical periodontal treatment, including scaling and root planing (a careful cleaning of the root surfaces to remove plaque and calculus (tartar) from deep periodontal pockets and to smooth the tooth root to remove bacterial toxins).

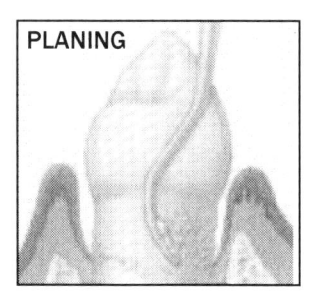

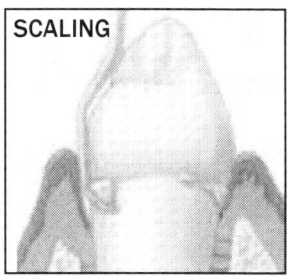

Most periodontists agree that after scaling and root planing, many patients do not require any further active treatment, including surgical therapy. However, the majority of patients will require ongoing maintenance therapy to sustain health. Non-surgical therapy does have its limitations, and when it does not achieve periodontal health, surgery may be indicated to restore periodontal anatomy damaged by periodontal diseases and to facilitate oral hygiene practices.

Regenerative Procedures

Procedures that regenerate lost bone and tissue supporting your teeth can reverse some of the damage caused by periodontal disease.

The periodontist you choose may recommend a regenerative procedure when the bone supporting your teeth has been destroyed due to periodontal disease. These procedures can reverse some of the damage by regenerating lost bone and tissue.

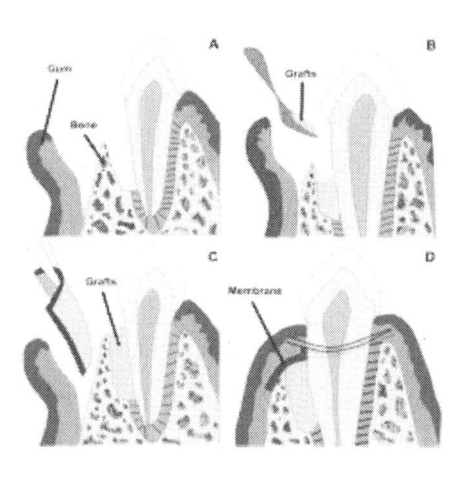

During this procedure, your periodontist folds back the gum tissue and removes the diseasecausing bacteria. Membranes (filters), bone grafts, or tissue-stimulating proteins can be used to encourage your body's natural ability to regenerate bone and tissue.

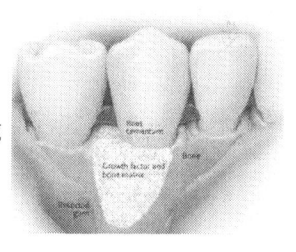

Eliminating bacteria and regenerating bone and tissue help to reduce pocket depth and repair damage caused by the progression of periodontal disease. With a combination of daily oral hygiene and professional maintenance care, you'll increase the chances of keeping your natural teeth—and decrease the chances of other health problems associated with periodontal disease.

Pocket Reduction Procedures

Your bone and gum tissue should fit snugly around your teeth like a turtleneck around your neck. When you have periodontal disease, this supporting tissue and bone are destroyed, forming "pockets" around the teeth.

Over time, these pockets become deeper, providing a larger space for bacteria to live. As bacteria develop around the teeth, they can accumulate and advance under the gum tissue. These deep pockets collect even more bacteria, resulting in further bone and tissue loss. Eventually, if too much bone is lost, the teeth will need to be extracted.

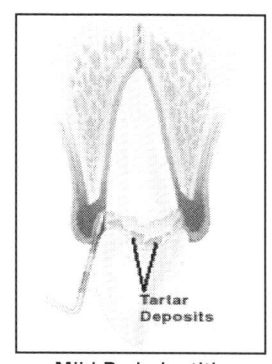

Mild Periodontitis 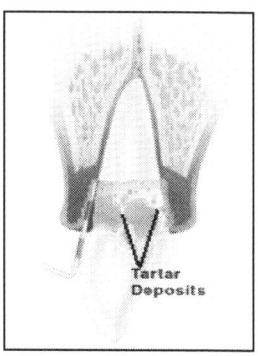   Advanced Periodontitis

Let's say the periodontist has measured the depth of your pocket(s) and has recommended a pocket reduction procedure because you have pockets that are too deep to clean with daily at-home oral hygiene and a professional care routine.

During this procedure, the periodontist will fold back the gum tissue and remove the disease-causing bacteria before securing the tissue into place. In some cases, irregular surfaces of the damaged bone will be smoothed to limit areas where disease-causing bacteria can hide. This will allow the gum tissue to better re-attach to healthy bone.

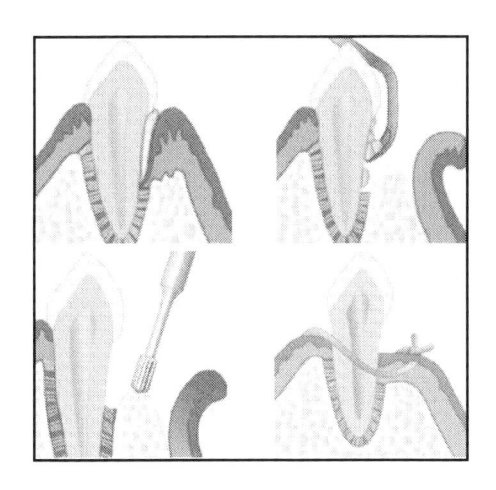

Reducing pocket depth and eliminating bacteria are important to prevent damage caused by the progression of periodontal disease and to help you maintain a healthy smile. Eliminating bacteria alone may not be sufficient to prevent disease recurrence. Deeper pockets are more difficult for you and your dental care professional to clean, so it's important for you to reduce them. Reduced pockets and a combination of daily oral hygiene and professional maintenance care increase your chances of keeping your natural teeth—and decrease the chances of serious health problems associated with periodontal disease.

Follow-Up Care

Why is follow-up necessary? I can't tell you how many patients I've consulted with over the past several years that have had periodontal treatment in the past but failed to stay on a regular follow-up or maintenance schedule. The disease was under control for a time, but eventually returned due to bacteria repopulation. Whether the recommended treatment is nonsurgical or surgical in nature, without follow-up care, the results will dissipate over time.

Research recommends that patients who have had periodontal treatment for gum disease follow a maintenance program every three months with their periodontist and/or dentist. Why? It takes roughly three months for the harmful bacteria involved with gum disease to repopulate a mouth after a cleaning. The theory is if a person has his or her teeth cleaned every three months, then the bacteria are not allowed to repopulate and cause continued destruction. Failing to follow a three-month maintenance program will not only cause gum disease to return, but it will also result in patients having to spend more money on additional procedures that may not have been necessary had they maintained their oral health.

> *"The patience and understanding that I have been shown both during and after my surgery have made all the difference in this experience. Thank you all very much."* — *Connie Frazier*

Chapter 5
The Photo Gallery
The Most Common Procedures: Pictures, Descriptions, & Questions

This chapter covers the most common procedures a periodontist performs, along with the recommended questions to ask about each type of procedure.

Free Gingival Graft

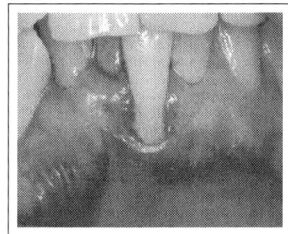

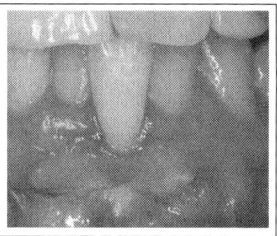

Before treatment   After treatment

The free gingival graft is used when more attached (hard) gingiva (gum tissue) must be added around the neck of a tooth. If there is inadequate attached gingiva, spontaneous recession of the gum and bone will occur over time. Typically the normal attached gingiva has been worn away with improper brushing, although some people are born with very little attached gingiva. When a new band of attached gingiva is created with a free gingival graft, the site becomes stable, and with proper brushing techniques, the results can be expected to last. It should be remembered that free gingival grafting is normally not performed to re-cover an exposed root.

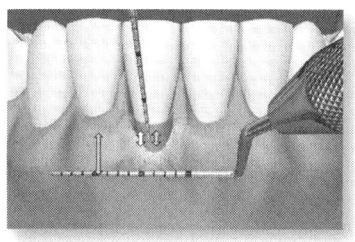

Gum recession and an inadequate amount of attached gingiva

What to Expect After a Free Gingival Graft

Have you ever burned your mouth by drinking hot coffee or eating hot pizza? If so, you have experienced what it feels like after a free gingival graft is taken from the roof of your mouth to be used for grafting. You should expect to use a medicated rinse to "numb" the palate or a clear stent to protect the palate after this type of graft. This procedure can be performed under local anesthesia, local anesthesia with sedation, or general anesthesia. After the rectangular-shaped graft is taken from your palate, a packing material is placed and the graft is secured with sutures that usually dissolve within a week or two. A packing material is placed around the graft to protect it from trauma while it is forming a blood supply. The packing material and any remaining sutures are removed at the two-week follow-up appointment.

Usually two or three follow-up visits are needed to assure that the graft forms a blood supply and survives the initial phase of placement. After three or four months, you should expect to be released back to your family dentist for regular care.

Questions to Ask If You Are Considering a Free Gingival Graft:

- How painful will the roof of my mouth be after surgery?
- Will the exposed roots be covered?
- When can I resume a normal diet?
- What happens if the graft does not "take"?
- I normally perform daily exercise. When can I resume this activity?

Connective Tissue Graft

When the gum has receded beyond the crown and the root is exposed, it is often desirable to re-cover the root surface. This is primarily done for cosmetic reasons, but it is also advisable if there is root sensitivity. There may also be a lack of attached (hard) gum tissue, and the root coverage surgery is designed to correct that problem at the same time.

Connective Tissue Graft

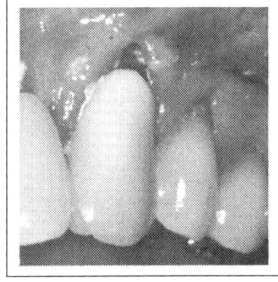

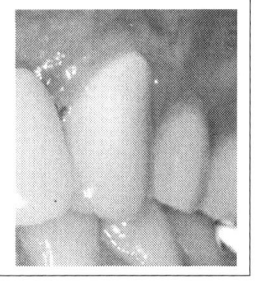

Before treatment   After treatment

What to Expect During a Connective Tissue Graft

During a connective tissue graft, the surgeon removes a thin piece of tissue from the roof of the mouth to provide a stable band of attached gingiva around the tooth. The graft may be placed in such a way as to cover the exposed portion of the root. The graft procedure is highly predictable and results in a stable, healthy band of attached tissue around the tooth. Your palate will feel similar to how it would if a free gingival graft had been performed (see above). A connective tissue graft can be performed under local anesthesia, local anesthesia with sedation, or general anesthesia.

Generally a packing material is not used for a connective tissue graft because the graft and the overlying tissue are sutured in place. The overlying tissue acts as an additional source of blood supply for the graft (the other source is the underlying tissue), and it also acts as a protective barrier. Follow-up care is similar to free gingival grafting.

Questions to to Ask If You Are Considering a Connective Tissue Graft:

- How painful will the roof of my mouth be after surgery?
- Will the exposed roots be covered?
- When can I resume a normal diet?
- What happens if the graft does not "take"?
- I normally perform daily exercise. When can I resume this activity?

"Before my treatment I was very concerned with pain during and after treatment. I was pleasantly surprised that the procedure was virtually painless! Dr. Anzalone's staff members are very friendly and knowledgeable, and their equipment is up-to-date and modern." — Ginger Graham

Dental Implants

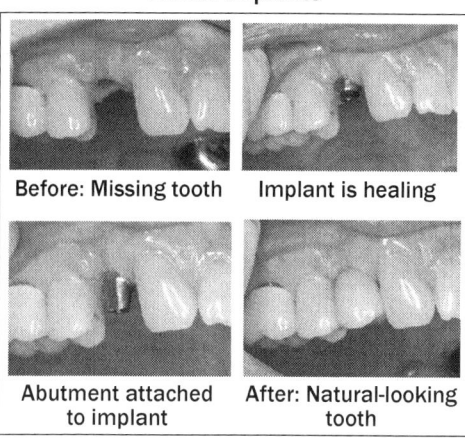

| Before: Missing tooth | Implant is healing |
| Abutment attached to implant | After: Natural-looking tooth |

Dental implants are designed to provide a foundation for replacement teeth that look, feel, and function like natural teeth. The person who has lost teeth regains the ability to eat virtually anything and can smile with confidence, knowing that teeth appear natural and that facial contours will be preserved. The implants themselves are tiny titanium posts that are placed into the jawbone where teeth are missing. The bone bonds with the titanium, creating a strong foundation for artificial teeth. In addition, implants can help preserve facial structure, preventing the bone deterioration that occurs when teeth are missing.

Dental implants are metal anchors that act as tooth root substitutes. They are surgically placed into the jawbone. Small posts are then attached to the implant, which protrudes through the gums. These posts provide stable anchors for artificial replacement teeth.

Implants are a team effort between a periodontist and a restorative dentist.

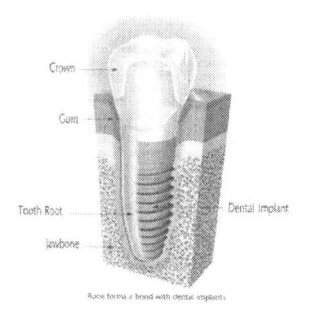

While the periodontist performs the actual implant surgery, as well as the initial tooth extractions and bone grafting if necessary, the restorative dentist (your dentist) fits and makes the permanent prosthesis (artificial tooth). Your dentist will also make any temporary prosthesis needed during the implant process to replace any missing teeth.

What to Expect During a Dental Implant Procedure

For most patients, the placement of dental implants involves one surgical procedure. Implants are placed within your jawbone. For the first two to three months following surgery, the implants are at the surface of the gums, gradually bonding with the jawbone. You should be able to wear temporary dentures or a partial if necessary, and you will eat a soft diet. During this time, your restorative dentist will design the final bridgework or denture, which will ultimately improve both function and aesthetics.

Questions to Ask If You Are Considering a Dental Implant:

- What can happen if I do not replace missing teeth with an implant?
- What is the main complication?
- How are implants inserted?
- How long have they been used?
- Are they safe?
- What are the chances of infection? What if this happens to me?
- If the implant has to be removed for any reason, can it be replaced later?
- Do implants break?
- How long does it take to heal?
- How do I know if I'm too old for implants?

Sinus Lift With Dental Implant Placement

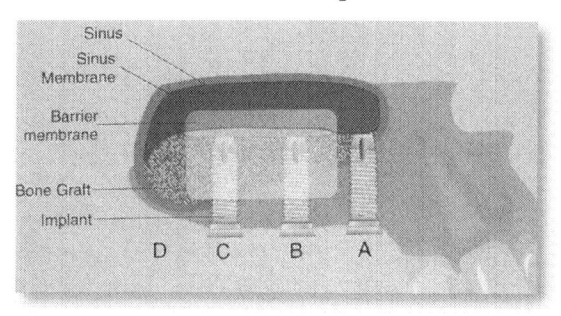

Usually the back three or four upper teeth reside either next to or inside the maxillary sinus. When a person needs a tooth removed and replaced in this section of the mouth, the sinus may need to be raised to make room for the implants. In the picture above, the classification of implant sites are labeled A through D.

Classification of Implant Sites
Class A: 10 mm or more of bone present under sinus
Class B: 7 to 9 mm of residual bone present under sinus
Class C: 4 to 6 mm of residual bone present under sinus
Class D: 1 to 3 mm of residual bone present under sinus
Class E: Absent or ablated sinus

Measurements can be taken on digital X-ray images that allow periodontists to measure the available bone under the sinus. Generally if a patient has 5 millimeters or more of bone under the sinus, an implant can be placed with a sinus lift. For those sites with less than 5 millimeters of bone, a separate sinus lift must be performed (discussed in the next section).

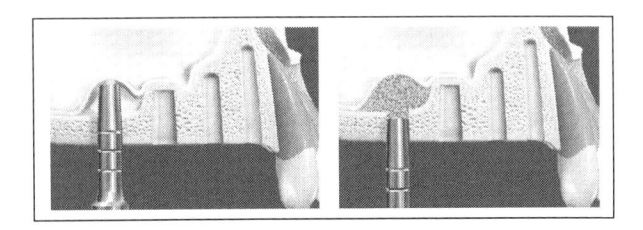

As you can see in the images above, the maxillary sinus can be gently raised using a series of special instruments. Once adequate height is obtained, bone is added to lift the sinus, followed by placing the implant(s). The bone acts as a natural "tent" to raise the sinus and also begins the process of the body forming new bone around the implant.

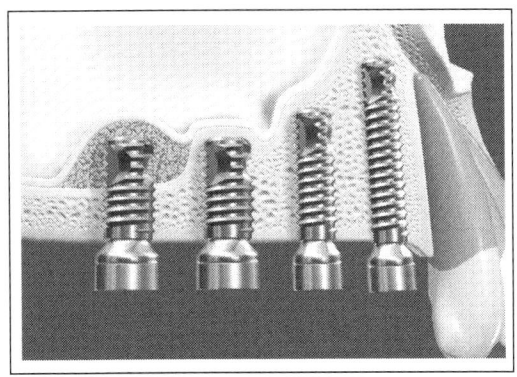

Implants placed after the sinus has been elevated

Sinus Lift as a Separate Procedure

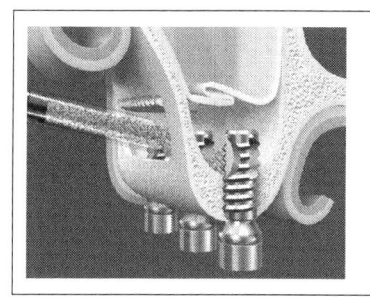

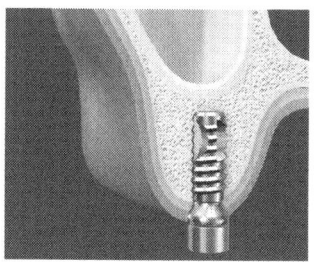

As discussed in the previous section, if less than 5 millimeters of bone is available under the sinus, a sinus lift is prescribed as a separate procedure. After local anesthesia is administered, the gum tissue is pushed back and a window is made in the front side of the jawbone adjacent to the maxillary sinus that needs modifying. Next, the sinus membrane is gently raised using special instruments, and a bone graft material is placed. Usually a resorbable membrane is placed over the opening, and the gum tissue is sutured closed. It usually requires six months of healing before an implant can be placed.

A sinus lift is one of the few procedures for which patients are usually placed on antibiotics and steroids before surgery to allow them to begin circulating in the bloodstream to decrease the chances of swelling and/or infection.

Sinus Perforation

The most common complication that can occur with sinus elevating augmentation is perforation of the sinus membrane. Research shows this complication can occur from 10 percent to 60 percent of the time. The membrane varies in thickness, but is generally only 0.3 to 0.8 millimeters.

A variety of techniques have been proposed to manage these perforations. These include using sutures, collagen membranes, fibrin sealants, or freeze-dried human bone sheets.

All these techniques involve repair of sinus membrane perforations that range in size from 2 millimeters to 1.5 centimeters. Typically a collagen membrane is placed over the perforation to prevent any grafting material from entering the sinus cavity. If the perforation is larger than 1.5 centimeters, the surgical site is closed and the body is allowed to heal (usually for two to three months) before entering the site again.

Researchers have noted a potentially helpful side effect of a sinus lift procedure. The ostium is a 7 to 10 millimeter long passage located at the top of the sinus that allows for drainage of fluids. Because the level of the sinus is raised, the distance the fluid in the sinus has to travel to reach the ostium is decreased, thus making drainage easier. I've actually had patients with persistent sinus trouble tell me the sinus lift procedure has eradicated their sinus issues!

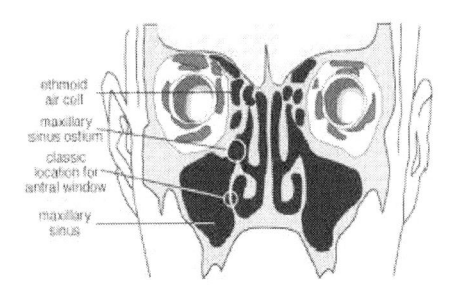

If you are considering a sinus lift procedure and have sinus trouble such as a chronic irritation, cysts, or polyps, it is imperative that you inform your periodontist. Usually a referral to a local ear, nose, and throat doctor is recommended to ensure the sinus is in good enough condition to be raised.

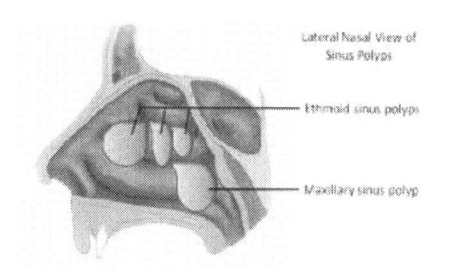

Lateral Nasal View of Sinus Polyps
Ethmoid sinus polyps
Maxillary sinus polyp

Questions to Ask If You Are Considering a Sinus Lift:
- What are some of the complications of the surgery
- What happens if there is a tear in the sinus?
- How long will the implants take to heal after they are placed in the grafted bone?

Bone Grafting

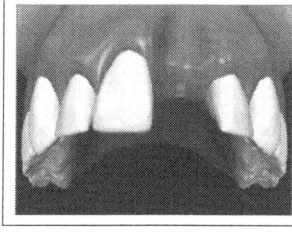

The tissues covering the bone will not hide the defect. Implant placement is not possible without bone grafting.

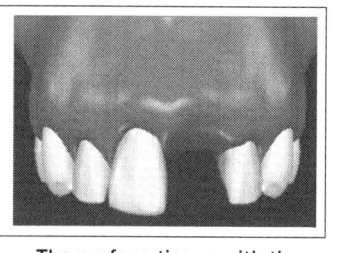

The surface tissue with the defect corrected.

When a patient has been missing a tooth for a long time, bone loss occurs. The picture on the left depicts a patient who had a front tooth removed several years ago and is now interested in replacing the tooth with an implant. Note the bone loss that has occurred by the indention in the gum tissue. After bone grafting to augment the site, note how the picture on the right now shows an extraction site that is ready for implant placement.

The Surgical Procedure
During the bone grafting procedure, the gum tissue is pushed away and a bone grafting material is added to the deficient area. Next, a resorbable membrane is placed over the graft. This membrane not only contains the material within the desired space, but it also prevents soft tissue from growing into the graft. Usually five to six months of healing is needed before reentering the site to place an implant.

Questions to Ask If You Are Considering a Bone Grafting Procedure:
- If I wear a temporary partial replacing the tooth, can I wear it after the procedure?
- Where does the bone come from?
- How long will my mouth be sore?
- How long does it take for the membrane to resorb?
- Can the implant and bone grafting be performed at the same time?

Esthetic Crown Lengthening

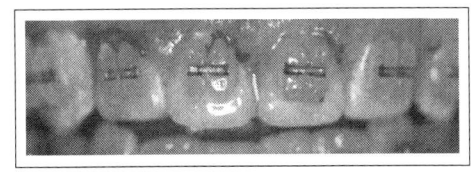

Before Treatment

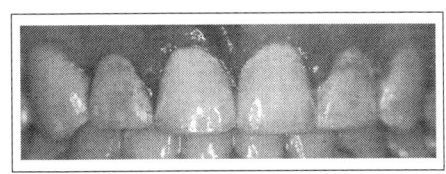

After Treatment

You may have wondered if there are any procedures to improve a "gummy" smile because your teeth appear short. Your teeth may actually be the proper length, but they're covered with too much gum tissue. To correct this, a periodontist performs an esthetic crown lengthening procedure.

> *Jenny's Story*
> *Even though Jenny was only 14 years old, she noticed that her teeth were much shorter than most of her friends' teeth. She asked her mom if something could be done to help, and her mom brought her in for a consultation. After reviewing all her options, Jenny's mom chose esthetic crown lengthening as the best option for her daughter, and she was amazed by the immediate transformation of her daughter's smile shortly after treatment.*

During the esthetic crown lengthening procedure, excess gum and bone tissue are reshaped to expose more of the natural tooth. Precise measurements of each tooth are taken beforehand to ensure the proper amount of tissue is removed. This can be done to one tooth or to several teeth to expose a natural, broad smile. The majority of the cases expose four or five teeth.

Questions to Ask If You Are Considering an Esthetic Crown Lengthening Procedure:
- How many teeth need to be lengthened?
- Does dental insurance sometimes cover this even though it is a cosmetic procedure?
- How long will it take for the gum tissue to heal?
- Will I need stitches?
- What happens if I need one or two teeth touched up in the future?

> *"I was concerned initially about the problems with my teeth, what could be done to them, and would gum treatment solve the problems. Everything was fully explained, and my concerns were gone. The treatment was performed excellently with continual concern for my comfort." — David Hage*

Crown Lengthening for a Restoration

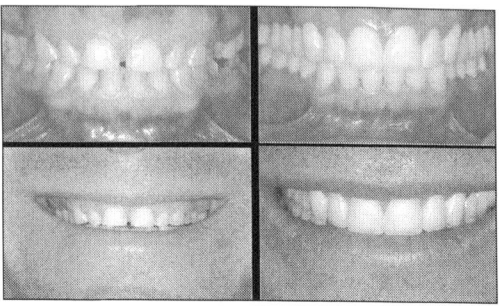

Before treatment   After treatment

Your dentist or periodontist may also recommend a dental crown lengthening procedure to make a restorative or a cosmetic dental procedure possible. Perhaps your tooth is decayed, broken below the gum line, or has insufficient tooth structure for a restoration such as a crown or a bridge. Crown lengthening adjusts the gum and bone level to expose more of the tooth so it can be restored.

Occasionally your dentist will send the periodontist a clear plastic guide that will fit over your teeth to show the periodontist the exact location where the gum tissue should be trimmed. Your dentist will make this guide by taking molds of your teeth and gums.

Questions to Ask If You Are Considering a Crown Lengthening Procedure for a Restoration:
- What can be done if the root is exposed after treatment?
- How long will I need to wait before my dentist can place the final restoration?
- What happens if the decay is too deep under the gum to restore the tooth?

"I was referred to Dr. Anzalone for dental extractions and dental implants. I was concerned about having pain after the procedures. I was given sedation during the procedures, and Dr. Anzalone did such a good job that I had NO PAIN afterwards. Dr. Anzalone was very informative and has a warm air of confidence about himself. I also appreciated Alice (his receptionist) calling me to remind me of the appointments."
— Julia Boddie

Tooth Extraction and Socket Grafting
Ridge Preservation - Bone and Membrane

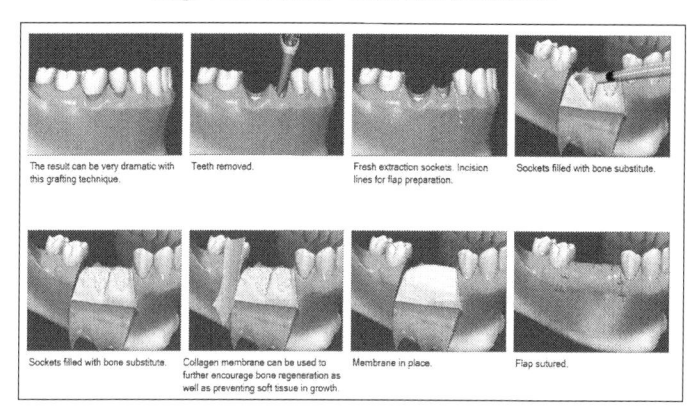

The result can be very dramatic with this grafting technique.	Teeth removed.	Fresh extraction sockets. Incision lines for flap preparation.	Sockets filled with bone substitute.
Sockets filled with bone substitute.	Collagen membrane can be used to further encourage bone regeneration as well as preventing soft tissue in growth.	Membrane in place.	Flap sutured.

There are times when teeth cannot be saved and have to be removed. Some of the reasons include decay, crown fracture, root fracture, abscess, and bone loss. After a tooth is removed, normal shrinkage of the bone will occur. The amount of shrinkage is unpredictable. Excessive shrinkage may prevent future placement of implants, create difficulty with your prosthesis, and compromise adjacent teeth or esthetics. It is common to place bone grafting materials into a socket immediately after the extraction of a tooth. This helps to maintain normal bone contours, and it significantly reduces the shrinkage of bone. The advantages are numerous: better implant base, support for adjacent teeth, improvement of aesthetics, and improved fit and function of your prosthesis.

Questions to Ask If You Are Considering a Dental Extraction and Socket Grafting:
- How long do I have to wait before an implant can be placed?
- How long does it take before the bone resorbs?
- Do the stitches dissolve?
- Can I wear a temporary partial to replace the missing tooth/teeth?

More Photos of Procedures
Connective Tissue Graft

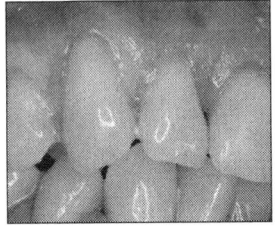

Before treatment 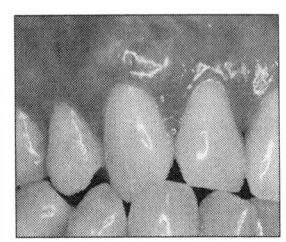 — After treatment

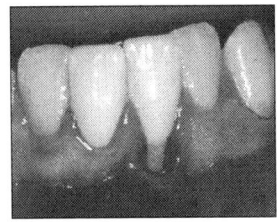

Before treatment 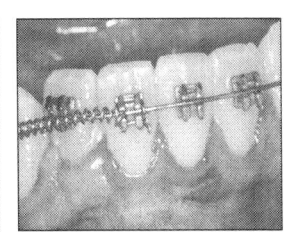 — After treatment

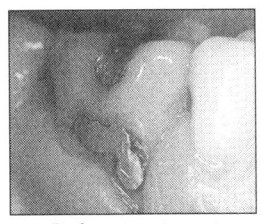

Before treatment 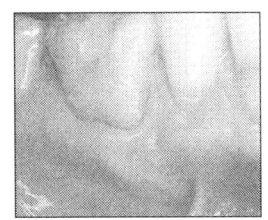 — After treatment

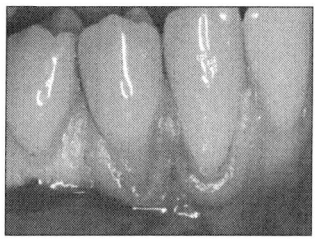

Before treatment 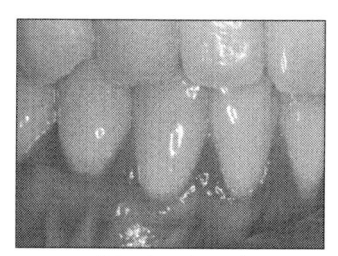   After treatment

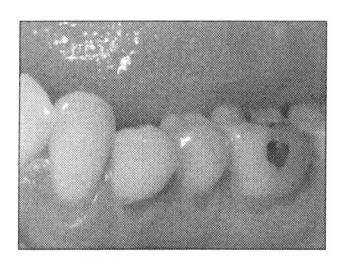

Before treatment 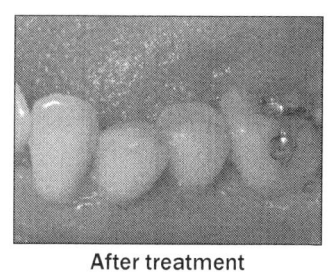   After treatment

Connective Tissue Graft + Crowns

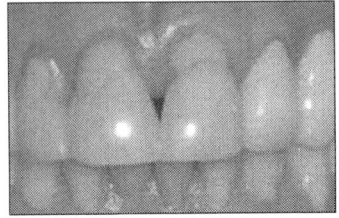

Before treatment

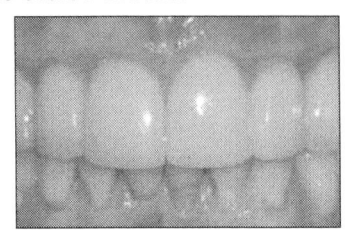

After treatment

Free Gingival Graft

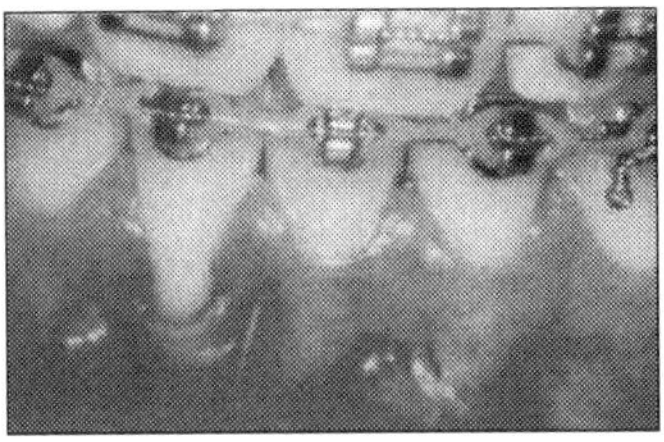

Before treatment

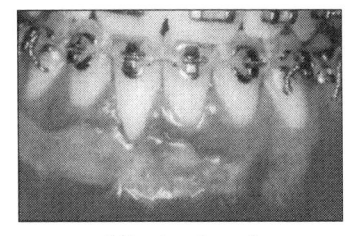

After treatment

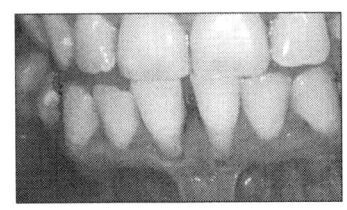

Before treatment

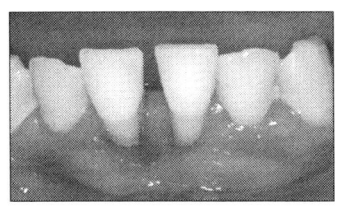

After treatment

Esthetic Crown Lengthening

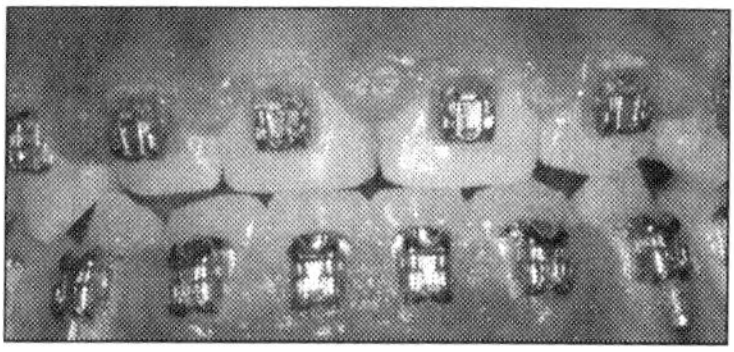

Before treatment

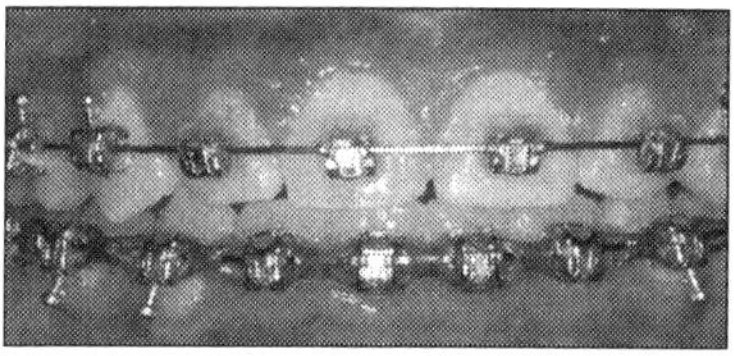

After treatment

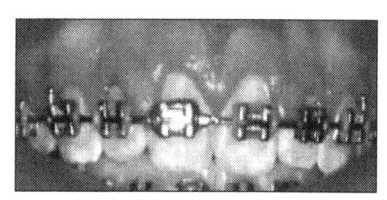

Before treatment

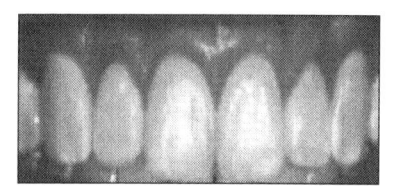

After treatment

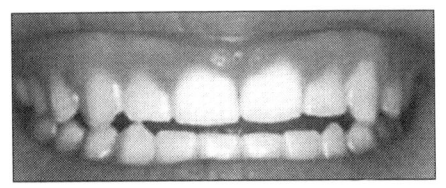

Before treatment

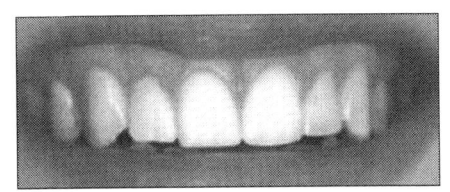

After treatment

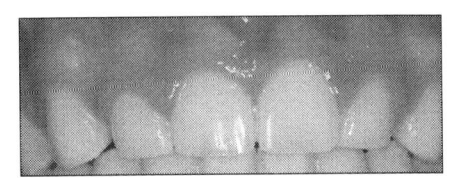

Before treatment

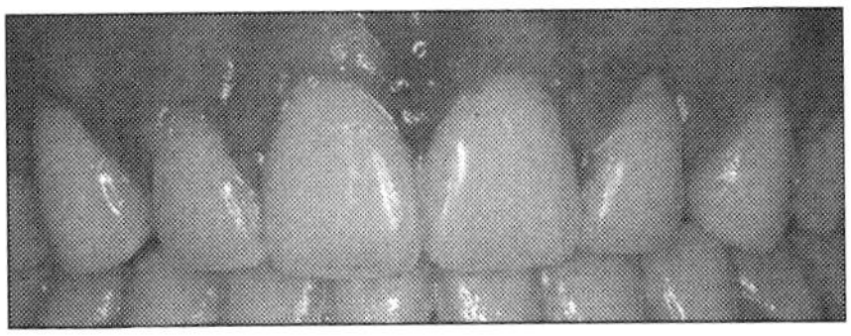

After treatment

Crown Lengthening for a Restoration

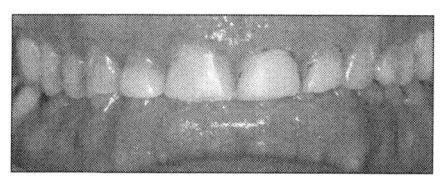

Before treatment

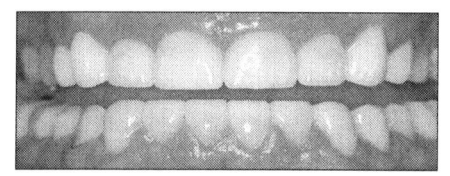

After treatment

Chapter 6
Dental Implants

What exactly are dental implants? Very simply put, dental implants replace the roots of teeth. They act as an anchor for crowns, bridges, dentures, or partials. They come in different lengths and widths in order to fit each individual's jawbone size.

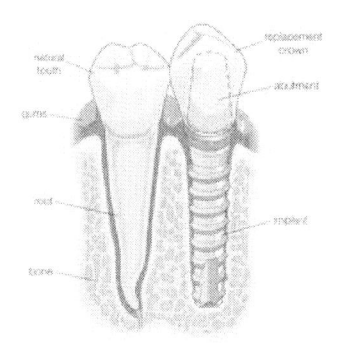

How are implants placed?

First, the surgeon administers a local anesthetic. If you have had a filling or other dental work, you will be familiar with the concept of "numbing." Next, the doctor makes an incision in the gum tissue on top of the area of the missing tooth. After the gum is pushed away, the surgeon prepares the bone by using a series of special drills that correspond to the size of the implant to be placed. Next, the doctor seats the implant and secures the gum tissue around the head of the implant with sutures.

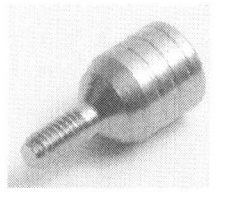

To complete the procedure, the dentist usually places a healing or protective cap over the top of the implant. This cap keeps food material from packing into the implant and also provides the gum tissue a platform on which to begin healing and shaping so it will match well with the surrounding tissue. Like implants, the healing caps come in different shapes and sizes to accommodate the height and thickness of a patient's gum tissue.

How long does it take for dental implants to heal?
Depending on the type of bone and a patient's situation, healing can take weeks to several months. Typical healing time is three to four months, but recently released technology can cut the healing time in half. Several factors will affect the speed with which a patient can put a new implant to use, such as the patient's age, density of the bone, location of the implant, and chewing function.

Increased Popularity
You may wonder why dental implants are becoming more popular. One of the biggest reasons is that dental implants give patients a permanent option for replacing missing teeth instead of using a bridge.

Bridge Versus Implant
You may be very confused at this point. Bridge? Implant? How is one to choose? Rest assured the answer to your question lies in your hands. First, let's discuss the definition of a dental bridge.

"I had to have false teeth on the top of my mouth. I went to my regular dentist who referred me to Dr. Anzalone because I couldn't keep my plate in. Dr. Anzalone put in implants, and now I don't have any trouble keeping my plate in and was real pleased with the results. I really liked him, and I really like his staff. I would recommend anyone to come to him because he's the best." — Bobbie Smith

Dental Bridge Just like a road bridge over a river "bridges the gap" from one side of the river to the other, a dental bridge "bridges the gap" created by one or more missing teeth. As you can see in this picture, a bridge is made up of two crowns for the teeth on either side of the gap—these two anchoring teeth are called abutment teeth—and a false tooth/teeth in between. The false teeth are called pontics and can be made from gold, alloys, porcelain, or a combination of these materials. While this has been a good restoration in the past, dentists are now shying away from recommending them. Why? The main reason is that with the success rate of dental implants, there is now NO REASON to cut down perfectly good teeth! (Placing crowns requires the dentist to grind down the natural tooth.) 106 Abutment teeth are prepared to receive crowns Patients with existing bridgework who get dental implants love the fact that they can clean and floss in between their teeth (implants) versus having to clean under the bridge. Food can pack under the bridge pontic, which can cause irritation and even decay under the bridge.

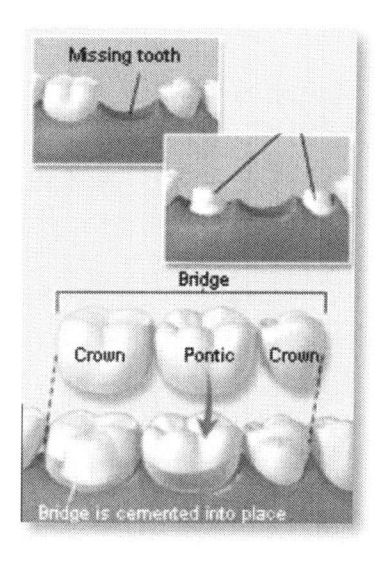

Patients with existing bridgework who get dental implants love the fact that they can clean and floss in between their teeth (implants) versus having to clean under the bridge. Food can pack under the bridge pontic, which can cause irritation and even decay under the bridge.

> ### Ben's Story
> *Ben came to our office after breaking off one of his front teeth. He was a successful professional, and he was very concerned about his appearance. The teeth on either side of the missing tooth were healthy. After discussing different treatment options to replace the missing tooth, Ben chose to replace his tooth with a dental implant. He informed me that he wanted something permanent, not removable, and he did not like the fact that with a traditional bridge, two healthy teeth would have to be cut down in order to replace one that was missing.*
>
> *Ben returned to see us after his implant was restored. He was very happy not only with the look, but with natural feel of his new tooth. He even told us his wife could not tell which one of his teeth was the implant!*

Repair or Replace?

Should an infected tooth be repaired, or should it be removed and replaced with a dental implant?

My patients ask me this question often. My answer to them is the same one I will give you here: It depends on the patient. Let me explain ...

Many things can cause a person to lose a tooth. Some reasons include decay, bone loss, infection, abscess, fracture (of the crown and/or root), failing root canal, and impaction, to name a few.

One of the main goals a periodontist should have for his or her patients is to save existing teeth whenever possible. If a tooth can be saved, I believe it is imperative to do so. When saving a tooth is a possibility, but the potential success rate is low, the periodontist and the patient should discuss the options. With today's technology, dental implant success rates are 90 to 95 percent at the 10-year mark. This success rate is making dental implants a very popular treatment choice.

Nancy's Story

Nancy's situation is one I encounter often. She had a root canal to treat decay that was causing her considerable pain. Root canal treatment involves removing the infected nerve of the tooth and placing root filling material within the empty nerve canal. This treatment worked very well for a period of years, but then Nancy noticed pain and a slight swelling around the gum tissue of the tooth. She returned to her family dentist, who had performed the root canal, and he believed the tooth was suffering from a gum and bone problem.

After examining Nancy's teeth, I thought the gum and bone loss around her infected tooth stemmed from an underlying gum disease problem associated with that tooth, or there was a chance the tooth root could be fractured.

Nancy was given two options:

1) have her dentist or an endodontist (root canal specialist) re-treat the root canal; or

2) have a periodontist remove the tooth, clean and graft the socket, and replace it with an implant.

Nancy had two concerns:

1) finances; and

2) she wanted a treatment that would definitely rid her of the infection.

Because of her express desires, I recommended removing her tooth, grafting the socket, and replacing the tooth with an implant.

What happens if I elect not to replace a tooth with an implant?
Once a tooth is removed, a series of events begins to take place. The body starts the process of forming new bone and gum tissue. As discussed previously, if bone grafting is placed in the extraction socket, this helps build a foundation for a future implant. If no grafting is placed, the jawbone begins to atrophy or shrink. A dental implant acts as a tooth root that supports the jawbone, and it also helps support adjacent teeth, preventing bone loss on each side of the implant.

Teeth can begin to shift as a result of not replacing a tooth with an implant. At times, the teeth behind and above the missing tooth drift into the space once occupied by a tooth. This can cause crowding of the teeth, and it changes the way a person bites.

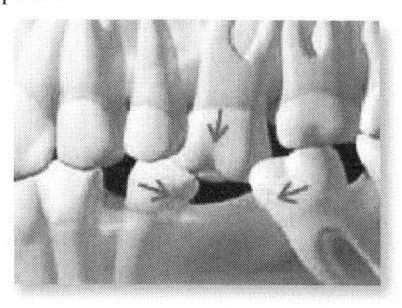

Sara's Story

Sara was a pleasant woman in her 60s who found our practice while researching dental implants online at our website, www.anzalone periodontics.com. She wanted to replace her back lower jaw teeth, which had been removed 15+ years ago. Sara was informed that because a considerable amount of time had elapsed since her extractions, her upper jaw teeth located above the missing teeth had dropped down to the point that they were nearly touching her lower jaw. Sara could tell that her upper teeth looked longer in the mirror, but she didn't know why. Unfortunately her upper teeth had to be removed and then replaced along with her lower teeth to correct her bite. The added expense of replacing her upper teeth could have been avoided if she had replaced her lower teeth in a timely fashion.

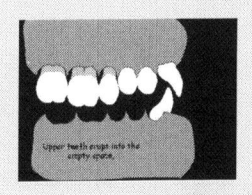

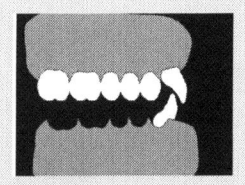

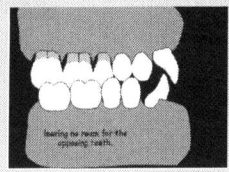

How many implants do I need if I'm missing several teeth?

A good rule of thumb is to place one implant per missing tooth. In some instances, two implants can be used as an anchor for a fixed bridge. The patient and the doctor should discuss all options on a case-by-case basis.

If a patient is missing all of his or her teeth, the periodontist should be able to recommend several options. The first question to ask is whether the patient would like a permanent, or fixed, restoration or something that is removable. This is the most important question to ask initially, because more implants are needed to support a fixed restoration versus a removable restoration.

Fixed Restoration

A fixed implant restoration is more costly than a removable implant restoration, and both your general dentist and your periodontist must work hand in hand during the entire treatment process. Generally a patient's dentist will indicate to the periodontist the location of the dental implants to support the fixed restoration. Models are fabricated by taking molds of the teeth and sending them to a dental lab. Next, a surgical implant guide is fabricated to help the surgeon place the implants in the exact location the dentist requests. Typically eight or more implants are used per jaw for a fixed restoration. Good home care and follow-up care are essential to ensure that the implants are being cleaned properly. Patients with fixed restorations are usually placed on a recall rotation with both the dentist and the periodontist.

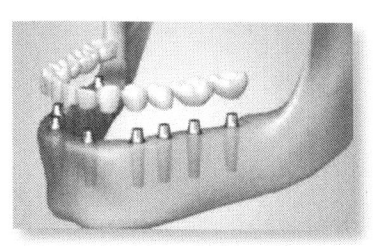

Implant Supported Restoration

Removable Restoration

Most patients who have an upper and a lower denture rarely complain about the top denture feeling "loose." This is generally due to the upper denture covering the entire roof of a patient's mouth, which causes suction for retention.

Sometimes patients request implants to hold their upper denture in place. These patients usually want to correct a sensitive gag reflex, or they want to be able to taste their food better. The entire middle section of the denture can be removed to correct these problems, as shown in these photos.

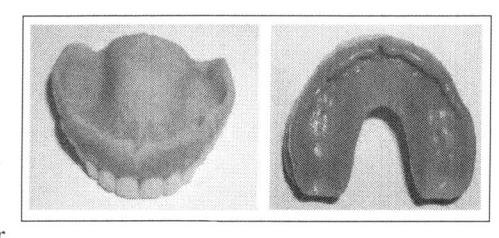

Most of the taste buds are on the tongue and the roof of the mouth. By removing the middle section of an upper denture, more of the patient's palate is exposed, thus allowing for a more natural sense of taste.

Denture wearers are more likely to complain of an uncomfortable and loose lower denture. This is due to the U-shape of the denture. Each time a person talks or chews food, the tongue and muscles of the cheeks move. This contraction and movement of the muscles can cause the lower denture to move.

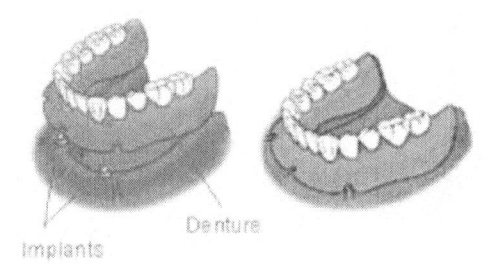

Usually patients who have a loose denture will either use glue or powder to help retain the denture. There's nothing worse than a denture falling out of someone's mouth while talking or eating. To avoid the possibility of being embarrassed, usually two to four implants can be placed in the front part of the lower jaw to help retain the denture. This allows the denture to be taken in and out and cleaned daily.

Can you be too young or too old to get implants?

That is a great question. Let's discuss being too young first. Girls typically stop growing between the ages of 16 and 17. For boys it is 18 to 21. During the growing phases, the jawbone grows, too. We typically wait until all growth is completed before placing implants. Usually a wrist X-ray can be taken and read by a radiologist to determine if the child's growth plates are fused and growth is completed.

I am often asked, "Am I too old for implants?" I have yet to read a study citing age alone as a determining factor for dental implants. Our office treats patients in their 80s and 90s with dental implants with very successful results.

> *Miss Betty's Story*
> *Miss Betty had worn dentures for over 30 years, and she had gotten to the point that she could not eat with them any longer due to discomfort and pain while chewing her food. As a result, she had lost a considerable amount of weight and was very unhappy. Miss Betty had learned about implants from a friend. She had many questions, but her main question was about her age (early 90s) and implants. She was told, as all of our elderly patients are told, that as long as a person is healthy enough to tolerate a procedure and there is adequate bone present, implants can be placed.*

Who benefits from having implants?
1. Current denture wearers who are fed up with the problems that can be associated with wearing dentures such as:
   - constantly using cream or powder to keep them in place
   - pain associated with chewing and talking
   - possibility of being publicly humiliated if teeth fall out during eating or talking
2. Patients who need to have teeth removed due to bone loss
3. Patients who need to have teeth removed due to decay or fractures
4. Accident or sports injury victims
5. Those with otherwise perfect teeth except for one or two missing teeth

Can I have dental implants if I have/had gum disease?
Even though the goal of every periodontist is to save a person's teeth, occasionally teeth have to be removed due to bone loss and mobility. If this happens, the teeth can be replaced as long as the gum disease is under control.

For patients who have recently had gum disease treatment, it is wise to wait at least six months before considering replacing teeth with dental implants around previously diseased teeth. The reason is it can take up to six months before the gum tissue and bone are fully healed and the periodontist can re-evaluate them to determine if the disease is under control. I know this may sound confusing, so let's walk through a typical example: John is referred to a periodontist to evaluate his gum disease that was recently diagnosed by his general dentist. After a thorough examination, the treatment plan is presented and accepted. John requires the removal of six teeth along with treatment of all of his remaining teeth for gum disease.

John goes to his periodontist's hygienist for regular cleanings at three months and then at six months after the gum disease treatment. During the six-month cleaning, his entire mouth is reprobed (rechecked) for resolution of the gum disease. Dental implants can be considered once this six-month checkup is performed and the gum disease is under control.

Bonus Section for Denture Wearers

Three Dangers of Tooth Loss and Poorly Fitting Dentures You Must Know About!

Danger #1: Bone Loss Makes You Look Older

Dental implants can help people look and feel younger because they prevent bone loss. By preventing bone loss that occurs with the loss of teeth, your facial structures remain normal and intact. The chances of wrinkling and looking old before your time are less likely. In other words, every day that you continue to wear dentures, you are experiencing bone loss—which makes you look older, as the pictures below illustrate:

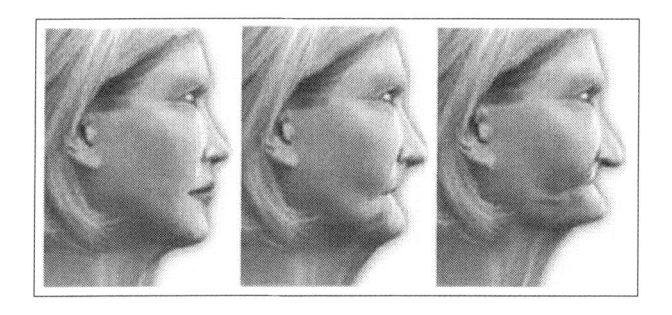

Danger #2: Poorly Fitting Partial Dentures Increase Your Risk of Tooth Loss and Gum Disease

When dentures don't fit properly, bacteria can get trapped in areas behind them and lead to gum and bone disease. Partial dentures that don't fit actually wear through the gum tissue and destroy the bone, causing loose teeth. The partial denture settles and the opposing teeth shift, making it even more difficult to chew. If a person with this problem waits too long, the treatment becomes more complex and can cost thousands of dollars more to fix.

Danger #3: Dentures May Reduce Your Life Span

It's true! Many people with poorly fitting dentures or multiple missing back teeth live shorter life spans (up to 10 years less) due to poor eating habits and stomach problems. They tend to eat more processed foods and experience many other health problems related to malnutrition. People now have options to dentures, and one of them is dental implants. People who get dental implants can finally eat the healthy foods they have been missing, such as apples, fresh vegetables, corn on the cob, and even steak!

Chapter 7
Sedation Dentistry

Secret: Know your options regarding sedation dentistry.

Can you guess the #1 question patients ask me daily? Maybe you've asked it, too: "Is my treatment going to hurt?" It's an important yet very easy question to answer. My answer is always a resounding "No." I can say "No" with confidence because of the many advancements the profession has made in sedation dentistry.

Do you fear going to the dentist? Rest assured, you're not alone. Some 75 to 80 percent of Americans experience feelings of anxiety about dental visits. In fact, roughly 25 million to 30 million Americans are deathly afraid of going to the dentist. But after you read this chapter that describes the different sedation options available, you will see that fear is really no reason to put off the dentistry treatment you may need.

The Difference Between Anxiety, Fear, and Phobia *(Source: www.dentalfearcentral.org)*
A distinction has been made between dental anxiety, dental fear, and dental phobia.

DENTAL ANXIETY is a reaction to an UNKNOWN danger. Anxiety is extremely common, and most people experience some degree of dental anxiety, especially if they're about to have something done that they have never experienced before. Basically it's a fear of the unknown.

DENTAL FEAR is a reaction to a KNOWN danger. "I know what the dentist is going to do, been there, done that—I'm scared!" This fear elicits a fight-or-flight response when the patient is confronted with the threatening stimulus.

DENTAL PHOBIA is basically the same as fear, only much stronger. "I know what happens when I go to the dentist—there's no way I'm going back if I can help it. I'm so terrified that I feel sick." This patient experiences the fight-or-flight response when just thinking about or being reminded of the threatening situation. Someone with a dental phobia will avoid dental care at all costs until either a physical problem or the psychological burden of the phobia becomes overwhelming.

What are the most common causes of dental anxiety, fear, and phobia?

Previous bad experience: In my opinion, this is by far the main reason for dental fear, ranging from anxiety all the way to a true phobia. We routinely ask our patients who have a severe form of dental phobia about when their problems started, and it usually stems from a bad past experience.

Humiliation: Occasionally we hear about dentists, hygienists, or staff members who may have made insensitive marks to patients. This can contribute to a dental fear.

Uncaring dentist: You might think that fear of physical pain is the main problem, but for some people it's actually emotional pain inflicted by a dentist who is perceived as cold and controlling. This can have a huge psychological impact.

What can help ease dental anxiety?

Dental professionals can use many things to help put a patient at ease, such as:

Relaxing environment

Hypnosis

Technology such as calming music

Communication—The way your dentist and his or her staff interacts with patients

Sedation/anesthesia

The remainder of this chapter is dedicated to discussing sedation dentistry.

Anesthesia Choices

Local anesthesia, also known as an "injection." Local anesthesia is needed for all dental surgery, whether or not sedation is used. The site to be treated must be "numbed" in order for a patient not to experience pain during and after the surgery is completed. The majority of the drugs used with IV sedation are not painkillers (although some are added occasionally). Most of the sedation medications are anti-anxiety drugs, which relax you. Inhalation sedation, also known as "laughing gas." Nitrous oxide is a gas that is breathed during treatment. After five minutes or so of breathing in the gas, patients usually experience a euphoric feeling that spreads throughout the body. Some describe it as a "happy drunk" feeling. Some people find there are auditory or visual effects as well. Patients will feel a bit lightheaded, and often people get "the giggles" (hence the name laughing gas). The main side effect is it can sometimes cause nausea.

IV (intravenous) sedation. With IV sedation, a drug to decrease anxiety is administered into the bloodstream during dental treatment. Different types of drugs can be used, with effects ranging from a state of total relaxation to deep sedation where the patient is actually asleep. Most of the drugs administered through the IV route cause amnesia (memory loss), which makes the treatment time seem to pass quickly.

How is IV sedation given?
"Intravenous" means that the drug is put into a vein. An extremely thin needle is put into a vein close to the surface of the skin in either the arm or the back of your hand. This needle is then replaced by a soft plastic flexible tubing through which the drugs are administered. The tubing is taped to your arm and stays in place throughout the procedure.

During the procedure, your pulse and oxygen levels are measured using a pulse oximeter. This gadget clips onto a finger and measures your pulse and oxygen saturation. It provides a useful early warning sign if you're getting too low on oxygen. Blood pressure before, during, and after the procedure should be checked with a blood pressure measuring machine. Most of these machines can be set to automatically take the blood pressure every four to five minutes during the procedure. Afterward, a printout of a patient's vital signs can be attached to the paperwork in the medical chart.

How safe is IV sedation? Are there any contraindications?

IV sedation is one of the safest types of sedation when carried out under the supervision of a dentist who has been properly trained. Each state dental board has specific regulations to which a dentist must adhere to perform sedation in his or her office. In Louisiana, certain education requirements are needed to obtain a sedation permit. A dentist must have a personal sedation permit (unless a medical doctor or a nurse anesthetist is administering the sedation) and an office sedation permit. The board will perform an on-site office inspection to make sure the appropriate emergency and monitoring drugs and equipment are present and that the dentist knows how to use them.

In addition to the above requirements, dentists seeking to use sedation must provide proof to the dental board of current certification in cardiopulmonary resuscitation (CPR) and advanced cardiac life support (ACLS). These requirements help to ensure the safety of patients who are to be sedated.

In addition to the safety afforded by proper training and regulatory oversight, the IV sedation process itself has certain "built-in" safety benefits. Due to the administration route (into a vein), drugs can be given in a precise manner to give the desired level of sedation for each patient. Several factors, such as drug tolerance and a patient's weight, determine the amount of medication needed. If problems arise, such as a patient's oxygen level becomes low or an allergic reaction is noted, the drugs can be reversed using reversal agents.

There are contraindications to sedation; some examples are: Pregnancy, a known allergy to sedation medications, and some instances of glaucoma.

Are there disadvantages?

Cost: IV sedation is more expensive than other sedation options. Recovery from IV sedation requires several hours after the dental procedure is completed. Drugs can "linger" in a person's system afterward, so a responsible escort is always recommended.

A hematoma (bruise) may develop at the site whre the needle enters the vein.

> *Mike's Story*
>
> *Mike had had a horrible experience as a child and this was the first time he had set foot in a dental office as an adult. He rarely smiled, was usually grumpy, and had lost self-confidence due to the many missing and decayed teeth in the front of his mouth. "It had been very difficult just to get him to come in for a consultation appointment," his wife, Sally, confided to me. I told her that both our office and his general dentist had a considerable amount of work to do to get Mike's mouth back into shape.; due to his previous dental experience, IV sedation was recommended.*
>
> *Mike's entire care took about eight months to complete, and he told me he is happier and\ smiles more than he has during any other time in his life. He was promoted at work and enjoys being out in public again. He attributes much of the success of his treatment to being able to fall asleep while the necessary dental treatment was being performed. I am very humbled to have been able to assist in Mike's "makeover."*

Chapter 8
Aftercare

Secret: Learning about "aftercare" before surgery will help decrease post-surgical complications.

Typical Recovery Times

Recovery after most periodontal procedures is usually prompt and uncomplicated. The majority of patients may return to their normal daily routines within a day or two. It's always best to take it easy the day of the surgery, and if you feel well the next day, you may resume normal activities.

What the Top Periodontists Do to Speed Your Recovery

With most businesses handing out less and less sick time each year, it's important to be able to return to work quickly after dental treatment. While once it was a matter of weeks before one could return to the office or school, today's periodontists speak of days, not weeks, to having you feeling "more normal" again.

Avoid the "4 Gs" - Garlic, Ginkgo, Ginseng, and Ginger. These and other herbal supplements can affect blood clotting.

Ensure adequate sleep - It is imperative that a patient gets seven to eight hours of sleep each night during the first two to three weeks after surgery. A proper sleep cycle is important for a speedy recovery and is usually disrupted if patients are in pain. The periodontist should provide proper pain medicine to help ensure this cycle.

Better pain control without the unpleasant side effects - If you have had trouble with pain medications in the past, please tell your periodontist ahead of time. The main side effect is nausea, and different medicines can be added to your prescriptions to stop pain in its tracks—all with minimal side effects.

Ensure a proper diet - The body needs protein to heal and fluids and carbohydrates to function normally. To ensure a proper diet while recovering, stock up on easily digested, soft foods that are high in proteins and moderate in carbohydrates. Protein smoothies are great, and they can be frozen and stored ahead of time. It's best to stick with soft, easy to digest foods the first two to three days post surgery. Examples include soups, bananas, Greek yogurt, wellcooked rice, and pureed foods. It's also imperative to avoid spicy, sticky, or crunchy foods because they can cause discomfort or damage to the recently treated area.

Other instructions - The cleaner you can keep the treated area after surgery, the better and more quickly you will heal—and with less discomfort. Your dental professional will give you detailed oral and written instructions after each procedure, because aftercare for each treatment is different.

> *"I was referred to Anzalone Periodontics for extractions and was concerned about the possibility of having pain with the procedure. Because of the explanation and pain management, I thought your office was great. We will recommend you to friends and family." — Eva Parker*

Chapter 9
Erasing Mental Blocks

Secret: There is a responsible answer for every concern or reservation about having dental surgery.

> *"I had very little pain after my procedure. The conscious sedation is my recommendation for procedures. I know that conscious sedation is the easiest way for treatment and that when you wake up the procedure is over. All other dental procedures were done using injections, and sometimes you still feel pain. This was the easiest procedure I have ever had done. I was very satisfied with Dr. Anzalone's treatment plan. He and his staff provided excellent care. I would highly recommend him to other people."* —Sue Street

If periodontal and dental implant surgery is as successful and as satisfying as it sounds, why isn't everyone having it done?
As we briefly touched on earlier, some patients have health conditions that prohibit treatment, under any circumstances. If this is the case, the patient will be told during the initial consultation that treatment is not possible.

Occasionally a patient's dentist will refer the patient to a periodontist to evaluate the need for treatment. Sometimes the patient does not need the requested treatment, may need non-surgical treatment, or may need a referral to a different specialist for evaluation.

I've found over my years of practicing that most prospective patients have the same reasons for putting off treatment. Below are the six most frequently stated issues and my honest responses:

"Will it be painful afterward?"
Each patient has a different pain tolerance, but most need nothing more than Motrin/Advil (ibuprofen) or a medium-strength pain medicine such as Lortab/Hydrocodone. You should be given these medications along with an antibiotic

if there is infection in the treated area or the potential for infection after treatment. The best dental practices are available 24 hours a day to ensure your comfort. Prior to surgery, be sure you are given a telephone number to reach the periodontist or one of the office staff members.

"I'm scared. The idea of having mouth surgery and sedation frightens me."

The majority of all periodontal procedures, like routine dental procedures, have few risks. Regardless of the procedure, you will be treated on an outpatient basis and will be able to leave the office very soon after treatment is completed.

"How long before I can return to work, social activities, or exercise?"

The majority of periodontal and dental implant procedures will not keep you from working or the things you enjoy doing for very long. We recommend that you take the day of the treatment off from school or work. You may return the following day. There are some exceptions with procedures that involve the entire mouth. These will be explained to you during the consultation.

"I read on the internet or had a friend tell me that this treatment doesn't work. Is that true?"

The internet contains a lot of good information, but it also contains information that is not reliable. Not a month goes by that at least one patient tells me the treatment was nothing like a friend or a relative had said it was going to be like. I guess the phrase "You shouldn't believe everything you hear" holds true.

"Can I afford the recommended treatment?"

Middle-aged men and women often tell me they need to put off their treatment so they can pay for their kids to go to college. Don't let money alone stand between you and your oral health. Postponing treatment will only worsen your condition, which ultimately will increase greatly the amount of treatment needed to bring your mouth back to health.

The top practices should offer multiple payment options, including interest-free financing. Whether or not a person has dental insurance, many of the needed services are either not totally covered or not covered at all. CareCredit is one of the most popular financing programs. It allows patients to spread their payments out for up to 60 months. Most practices can call the finance companies for you, or you can fill out a form online and know whether or not you qualify within minutes.

"Which doctor is best qualified to treat me?"
Following the guidelines in this book should help you make the right decision. The most critical factor is to choose a periodontist who has the proper experience and qualifications and with whom you feel comfortable and confident of a good outcome. Surgical outcomes are directly related to the experience, skill, and degree of specialization of the practitioner.

Chapter 10
The Relationship Between Your Dentist and Your Periodontist

Some patients find their way to a periodontist's office by doing research on the internet. Others receive a recommendation from a family member or a friend. But most patients are referred to a periodontist by other dentists.

Why can't my dentist treat me?

Dentists are not all the same. Some choose to focus their practices on procedures that interest them, such as cosmetic dentistry. Most of the dentists from whom our practice receives referrals choose not to treat gum disease surgically or to place implants surgically in their offices. When a dentist limits his or her practice to the specialty for which he or she has trained, that dentist only performs procedures within that chosen scope of practice.

This is not the case for a general dentist. General dentists can perform any type of treatment for which they have been extensively trained.

Can my dentist treat my gum disease?

Yes, if he or she chooses to. Most general dentistry practices employ one to three dental hygienists. One of their responsibilities is to treat gum disease non-surgically. A hygienist can begin the process of eliminating gum disease with scaling (removing plaque at and just below the gum line) and root planing (deep cleaning). If a hygienist does not choose to perform scaling or root planing, or when the gum disease is severe, often the hygienist will make a recommendation for the patient to see a periodontist for an evaluation. The dental practices with which we work do a fabulous job of recognizing, treating, and/or referring patients regarding gum disease. Because of this strong partnership, our patients feel at ease and trust their dentists' and hygienists' decisions on when to treat and when to refer.

Why do I have to go to another office for an implant?

We often are asked this question, and it's a great one. As stated before, the majority of general dentists do not place implants, even though they are capable of doing so. They simply choose not to do this procedure. When this is the case, these dentists refer patients to a periodontist and the consultation process begins.

Generally a patient can expect a three to four month healing period after receiving implant treatment before returning to his or her dentist to have the tooth restored. The office that places your implant should make you feel as comfortable as your dentist does. You should think of your periodontist's office as a "home away from home." If you are not comfortable with a periodontist or the plan of treatment, ask your dentist for other periodontists' names so you can get a second opinion.

Restoring your mouth to good health should be a positive experience. If you follow the recommendations in this book, you will be able to make confident decisions about your oral health that will pay you health dividends for the rest of your life. So, don't wait. A healthy smile is waiting for you!

Made in the USA
Columbia, SC
20 June 2023